Praise for *The Big Book of Magi*

Mastros's *Big Book of Magical Incense* is so much more. Sara's personal experiences, scholarship, insights, and observations make this book a guide to deepening your understanding of the many uses for incense. There are also many wonderful recipes, but more importantly, the rationales for the recipes are explained and ritual practices for their use are shared. *The Big Book of Magical Incense* is more than a reference book, it is an enjoyable read, as well, that you will return to many times."

—Ivo Dominguez Jr., author of *The Four Elements of the Wise*

"Sara Mastros has written the guide to magical incense I wish I'd had forty years ago when I was a baby Witch. Her *Big Book of Magical Incense* is exceptionally well-organized and well-written, and there is an extensive bibliography. Experienced practitioners will find this book useful in many types of magical operations, while beginners will discover a wealth of information on every page."

—Caroline Kenner, former owner of The Fool's Dog e-Tarot, emerita organizer of Sacred Space, and Washington Witchdoctor

The
Big Book of
Magical
Incense

SARA L. MASTROS

WEISER
BOOKS

For my beloved and ever-dependable Muses:
you know who you are.

This edition first published in 2021 by Weiser Books, an imprint of
Red Wheel/Weiser, LLC
With offices at:
65 Parker Street, Suite 7
Newburyport, MA 01950
www.redwheelweiser.com

Copyright © 2021 by Sara L. Mastros

ISBN: 978-1-57863-740-9
Library of Congress Cataloging-in-Publication Data available upon request.

Cover and interior design by Kathryn Sky-Peck
Cover photograph Olivier Rapin Photographie/Getty Images
Typeset in Times New Roman

Printed in the United States of America
IBI
10 9 8 7 6 5 4 3 2 1

THE PRACTICES IN THIS BOOK involve plants, toxins, and techniques that may be dangerous or fatal if used or performed improperly. Every effort has been made in the text to encourage the practitioner to use proper safety precautions in the rituals and recipes. This book also contains advice and information relating to herbs and is not meant to diagnose, treat, or prescribe. It should be used to supplement, not replace, the advice of your physician or other trained healthcare practitioner. If you know or suspect you have a medical condition, are experiencing physical symptoms, or feel unwell, seek your physician's advice before embarking on any medical program or treatment. Readers using the information in this book do so entirely at their own risk, and the author and publisher accept no liability if adverse effects are caused.

Contents

Part One
Fundamentals

How to Burn Loose Incense • Making Oils from Loose Incense •
Making Baths from Incense

Cones • Sticks • Cigars

Part Two
Ingredients

Part Three
Recipes

Part One

Fundamentals

How to Use This Book

WELCOME TO *The Big Book of Magical Incense*. I'm excited to be able to share it with you. I had two goals in writing this book. The first is simply to share my personal recipe book of incenses I use in my own life and witchcraft. More importantly, however, I'd like to help you develop your own incense practice. To that end, we'll begin by very briefly discussing the power of scent and the history of how humans have harnessed that power in incense. From there, we'll investigate the craft of incense making. Of all potion forms, loose incense is probably the simplest to make. Because of this, it's a great place to start learning about magical materia. Most of what you learn about incense will carry over directly into many other types of witch's crafts, as well as into the practical sorcery we call witchcraft.

Because the goal of this book is to give you the knowledge you need to experiment, instead of jumping right into recipes, we'll first take some time to really study the ingredients used in incense. We'll discuss more than fifty ingredients from which you can make incense, focusing on those that are easy to grow, wildcraft, or find in your local grocery store. As we do, we'll talk about how to make choices and substitutions based on your own pantry. To that end, I've organized the materials into categories. Of course, this book doesn't—nor could any book possibly—cover *all* the ingredients that can be used to make incense. Instead, this book will provide you with the tools to understand any ingredient and, by analyzing its chemical and cultural properties, grasp its magical uses as well.

Next, you'll learn more than sixty individual recipes for incenses of many different types. You'll see incenses designed to delight the senses and carry the imagination to fantastical realms. You'll learn offering incenses for many, many kinds of spirits, including ecoregional nature spirits, gods, demons, and your own ancestors. The focus will always be on understanding why those particular ingredients were chosen and how they come together to form a coherent whole. Examples are chosen to show the widest possible variety, so you can mix and match them to suit your own needs. Many of these recipes are accompanied by spells, both ancient and modern.

Once we've mastered offering incenses, we'll move on to incenses designed to accompany specific types of spells, often called condition formulas. You'll learn magic to cover all the bases. We'll discuss both ethereal and mystic types of magical incense, like Oracle's Smoke or incense to bless tarot cards, as well as very practical concerns goals, like attracting lovers or making bad neighbors move away.

After seeing my recipes, we'll examine in detail some ancient recipes, such as kyphi and ketoret. From those examples, you'll learn how to adapt other historic recipes for modern use. Historic recipes, even when they are complete and comprehensible, often include unidentifiable or practically/ethically unobtainable ingredients. Because the modern recipes I am offering are all my own creations, I can explain in great detail why I chose each ingredient. Using those examples, we'll try to tease apart why these ancient recipes might be constructed the way they are. Once we understand that, we'll learn how to reconstruct partially or completely lost recipes.

In addition to the incense itself, I've tried to use examples of spells and rituals from many different styles of practice, while still providing a holistic approach. In this book, you'll see spells from the ancient Greek Magical Papyri next to early 20th-century American folk magic, elaborate Solomonic invocations as well as rhyming cantrips to share with your children and house spirits. One of my goals with this book is to provide you with a sampler from which you can branch out and research those things that most kindle your interest. My greatest hope is that your time with this book provides both a solid grounding in the fundamentals, as well as the confidence and inspiration to adapt, improvise, and experiment to create your own incense practices. This book isn't intended for your library, but for your laboratory, where you get your hands dirty and try things.

This book is not intended to serve as an academic reference nor as an unbiased account of a body of factual information. Such sources are already both various and ubiquitous; many of them are listed in the bibliography. Moreover, in today's rapidly evolving information landscape, books are not appropriate vessels for that type of encyclopedic compendia, which are far better served by hypertext media. Books, as a medium, are best when they are intimate communication between reader and author, and that is how I urge you to approach this book: not as a conversation with incense, but as a conversation with me.

This is an extremely biased and heavily curated tour through my personal relationship with that body of knowledge and a guided apprenticeship in the practical craft of using that body of knowledge. While I have attempted always to truthfully communicate to you my best understanding of the facts at hand, I am sure that many of the authors I have cited would fundamentally disagree with the conclusions I have drawn from their work and with the rhapsodic recontextualization in which I have engaged. The only authority I am appealing to in this book is my own, and the only appropriate way for you to verify if what I say is true is experimentally, by building your own relationship with incense—not just in your mind, but in your hands and in your nose—and by engaging in your own conversation with the plants, spirits, and procedures I am talking about. This book is not a work of scholarship, it is a game of scholarship, and one I hope you will enjoy playing with me.

The Science of Scent

SCENT IS ONE of our most primal senses; our deepest ancestors first learned to smell more than half a billion years ago.[1] Scent is the only sense that completely develops in the womb; our ability to smell is fully formed by the end of the first trimester.[2] Scent is also the only sense to pass through the amniotic fluid.[3] Throughout the rest of a pregnancy, the fetus smells everything the mother smells.[4] This is why fretful newborns can sometimes be quieted by being wrapped in their mother's clothing. Some speculate this is why newborns appear to emerge from the womb already recognizing their family*; they've already smelled them in utero.[5]

Smelling is a fascinating process. Tiny particles in the air pass through a layer of mucus at the back of the olfactory cavity and directly interact with a small piece of the olfactory bulb, which extends outside your skull, high in your nasal cavity.[6] There, the particles "fit into" specialized smell receptors, of which we have about four hundred different kinds.[7] Those forty different receptors can be thought of as primary scents in a way similar to the three primary colors. Most humans can discern about a trillion distinct smells. For comparison, human eyes have only three different types of receptors, which allow us to see approximately ten million distinct colors.[8]

Unlike sight, where we can easily see and understand a whole vista of many complex sights at once, we smell everything in our environment as one jumbled-up scent. Most people can distinguish only about three

---

* Following ancient custom, throughout this book the word *family* includes everyone you live with, whether or not they are genetic relations.

distinct smells before they lose their ability to tell them apart.[9] However, with training, humans can learn to pick apart much more complicated smells. Most modern commercial perfumes contain around four hundred individual scent-bearing molecules, and well-trained perfumiers can identify all of them.[10]

Some people believe that scent is somehow more subjective than our other senses, but that is not true. Smell provides us with factual information about our immediate environment; it is just as objective as sight or hearing. While it's certainly the case that the sense of smell is deeply entwined with memory, much of this sensation is not dependent on memory.[11] While many of us associate the smell of vanilla with childhood treats, that is not what makes the smell pleasant. The chemical constituents of vanilla calm anxiety not just in humans who remember cupcakes, but in many other nonhuman animals as well.[12]

Like taste, smell involves taking small pieces of our material environment directly into our body. For that reason, smells can impact our emotions without having to pass through the filter of our rational mind. Scents are drugs. For example, birch tar, jasmine, lavender, and lemon have all been shown to increase theta brain wave (calming) activity, even in subjects who reported different subjective responses to those odors.[13] Rosemary increases frontal alpha waves (increasing alertness, memory, and focus) and decreases beta waves (which are correlated with drowsiness).[14] Although clearly not an unbiased source, one Japanese fragrance marketer claims that typos and other typing errors decrease up to 54 percent when offices smell of lemons.

Today, many corporations develop carefully tailored signature scents with which they infuse stores and working environments to produce behaviors they desire. For example, SoulCycle gyms have a trademark smell, which to me seems mostly like grapefruit with undertones of lemongrass and ylang-ylang. While that kind of sophisticated manipulation is out of the reach of many mom-and-pop shops, research indicates that even a simple orange scent in a store can increase per-customer spending by up to 20 percent.[15] These physiological effects are one of the cornerstones of the magical use of scent.

We are often told that humans have a very poor sense of smell compared to other animals, but that is simply not true. Mice, for example, can smell many things that humans cannot, but humans can smell many things in much weaker concentrations than mice can, although rats and dogs can smell most things at lower concentrations than humans.[16] However, some scents—such as human blood—are more easily detected by humans than even dogs.[17] When humans are blindfolded and asked to follow a smell trail on their hands and knees like a dog, we do remarkably well. For some smells, particularly florals, many humans outperform untrained dogs. Many scientists believe that the almost universal human behavior of kissing may have evolved as a way to smell and taste a potential mate, just like dogs sniff each other's butts.[18] However, a century of bad science, rooted primarily in the idea that humans are too "rational" to be led by our sense of smell, has until recently convinced many of us that we shouldn't even bother trying to investigate our environment with our sense of smell.

Different people have different olfactory abilities. Some components of smell sensitivity are genetic. Broadly speaking, women are better at smelling than men are, and pregnant women are especially sensitive to smells. Several diseases can interfere with our ability to smell, either temporarily or permanently. All humans lose our sense of smell as we age, starting slowly in the early thirties, with a more precipitous decline in old age. However, there are many things you can do to improve and safeguard your sense of smell; the most important is to quit smoking. Long-term smokers are more than six times as likely to report problems with their sense of smell as nonsmokers. You can also use an air filter in your home, especially if you live somewhere with poor air quality like I do.

However, the most important feature of smell training is practice. As you go through your day, take the time to identify what you are smelling. Name the individual scents. Make a point every day to smell several strong scents, like fruits, spices, coffee, soaps, herbs, and flowers. As you practice, try to smell them from farther and farther away. Once you've learned to identify a particular scent, start to practice imagining it. Get a partner, and quiz each other at identifying different smells. Once you're good at that, start mixing scents for your partner to identify. Start with just two at a time and work your way up to more.

If you want to get serious about scent training, you can buy sets of essential oils designed for just this kind of practice. Those are great for people who've damaged their sense of smell and need very strong scents to train with, but for most people, I think you're better off practicing with whole ingredients, which have subtler and more complex scents, instead. Each time you smell a particular scent, the synapses involved in producing that scent sensation are strengthened. That means that the next time you smell it, you'll be able to detect it at a lower concentration. Moreover, each new thing you smell helps you build a mental library of scents you can compare against new smells to help identify them.

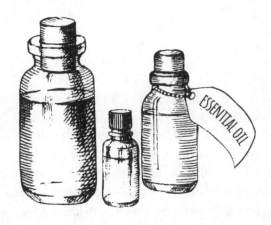

A Very Brief History of Incense in the West

MATERIALS BURNED primarily for their scent are difficult to detect in the archaeological record exactly because incense is defined by its intended use, rather than its actual composition. As you'll see over the course of this book, many incense ingredients are also culinary and medicinal materials. Therefore, it's difficult to be sure how humans used them before the advent of writing. For example, balls of sweet-smelling resins are found at many prehistoric sites,[19] but there's no way to know if they were used as incense, as medicine, as a food flavoring, as a glue, or any other potential purposes. I am no archaeologist, but to me it seems that it couldn't have taken long for humans who had mastered fire to learn that some things smell better than others when burned, so I assume basic incense* was a very, very early human invention.

By the third millennium BCE, the ancient cultures of China, the Indus Valley, Mesopotamia, and Egypt all had sophisticated incense practices and participated in a complex web of trade in incense ingredients. Myrrh, frankincense, cinnamon, cassia, jasmine, spikenard, and sandalwood were all popular incenses, both individually and in mixed recipes. The earliest known records of the incense trade are from Egypt, where the Eleventh Dynasty (3580–3536 BCE) king Assa (Tet-ka-ra) sent an expedition through the desert in search of frankincense.[20] The Egyptian lust for incense

---

* That is to say, biological material burned solely for its smell.

grew truly insatiable over time. It is said that Ramses II (1279–1213 BCE) received 368,461 jars of incense as tribute in his thirty-year reign.[21]

By the mid-second millennium BCE, a flourishing and well-established trade network, often called the Incense Road, linked the Mediterranean, Africa, Arabia, and India. In addition to frankincense, myrrh, and other precious resins and incense spices, traders also offered pearls, gems, and precious metals, along with silks and other textiles, ebony and other precious woods, and all manner of luxury items. However, perhaps the most important things traded along the Incense Road were ideas and stories; cultural diffusion along these trade routes played a major role in helping to create what we now call Western civilization.

As so often happens, tensions over control of this trade sometimes erupted into war. For example, the Syro-Ephraimite War of the 8th century BCE described in the biblical Book of Isaiah was almost certainly fought at least partially over control of the northern portion of the Incense Road.[22] The desire for incense was among many reasons Alexander of Macedon set out to conquer Arabia. In Book XII of his *Natural History*, Pliny tells a humorous story that, as a child, Alexander was reprimanded by his tutor Leonidas for being wasteful with frankincense on his altar. He was told that when he conquered the incense lands, he might use as much as he liked. The story goes on to say that, when Alexander conquered Arabia, he sent Leonidas a ship full of frankincense, with a message not to be so cheap with the gods.

By the 1st century BCE, the Roman Empire controlled most of the incense trade in the region, and direct trade between Rome and India became more common. However, beginning in the 3rd century CE, widespread economic decline across the empire led to a sharp dip in the importation of incenses. This caused economic decline and strife in the incense-producing nations of the Arabian Peninsula and the rise of the Himyarite kingdom. Back in Rome, the widespread adoption of Christianity was another blow to the incense trade; the early Patriarchs forbade the use of incense in worship as a pagan practice.

The first well-documented Christian application of incense was at the funeral of St. Peter of Alexandria, in 311 CE.[23] By the late 4th century CE, incense was in widespread use in the Eastern church and slowly spread through the Western church as well. In 735 CE, the famed scholar

Bede the Venerable was about to die. A fellow monk at the monastery of Monkwearmouth-Jarrow in Northumbria named Cuthbert tells us Bede asked to distribute his possessions, saying, "I have a few treasures in my box: some pepper, and napkins, and some incense. Run quickly and fetch the priests of the monastery, and I will share among them such little presents as God has given me." From this, we can ascertain that, while incense was becoming more available in Western Europe, it was still very precious.[24]

In the 14th century, with the invention of sophisticated alcohol extraction techniques, perfumery began to diverge from the more general incense, oil, and aromatics craft. This made possible the development of light, ephemeral, floral scents that cannot be captured in (non-synthetic) incense. Around the same time, incense rose to prominence in Japan, where it blossomed into an elaborate art form called *kōdō*, or "the way of fragrance." This led to a creative explosion in incense creation, and many new forms and recipes were developed.

With the European conquest of the Americas, many new plants and incense practices were introduced into the Western incense tradition. By the late 17th century, many incense makers were turning away from natural ingredients in favor of the synthetics coming out of the perfume industry industry. *Kōdō*-style incenses were introduced into the Western scent vernacular at the 1893 Chicago World's Fair, and those too were soon available in synthetics. Today, synthetic scents are a $4.2 billion-dollar industry, but there are still those of us who prefer scent in its most primitive form: incense.

How to Prepare & Use Loose Incense

THE MOST IMPORTANT step in making incense is to decide what sort of incense you want. Conveniently, most of this book will be dedicated to that topic! The recipes here are intended as examples, not gospel. This isn't chemistry, it's art. Natural products will always vary from one harvest to another. Unless you are using 100 percent synthetic materials, it is impossible to be precise in your incense making even if you try. All recipes in this book are measured by volume, not by weight, but except when I'm testing recipes for you, I don't really measure at all.

Once you've decided on your recipe, it's simply a matter of grinding and mixing. I strongly recommend an electric coffee grinder, but you can also grind by hand with a mortar and pestle. Freezing resin before powdering makes it easier to grind. Whatever you use, you'll want to dedicate that tool to magical use and not use it for food preparation. Ground resin is very difficult to fully clean, so you should expect some amount of cross contamination between everything that goes through that grinder. How finely you grind your ingredients is up to you. Finer ground incense will produce a lot of smoke very fast; larger chunks will last longer. For most purposes, I like to have multiple sizes in each incense, so the smell subtly unfolds and changes over time.

Particularly if an incense has ingredients of different densities—like dried herbs mixed with resin—you'll probably want to use something sticky to bind it all together. I like to use honey, which imparts its own warm and sweet scent to the mixture. Before adding the honey, reserve about 10 percent of the dry incense. Add just enough honey to the rest to get it to stick together. If you put in too much honey, add the reserved powder back in. Burn a small pinch of the ground incense. Are you happy with how it smells? If not, combine a pinch of this and a dash of that and keep testing until you are. Open your inner senses and allow intuition to guide you. You know how, sometimes, you might have the munchies, and you stand in front of the refrigerator until something calls out to you? That's also a good way to choose the variables in your mix.

Once you're happy with the incense, you can either burn it right away or let it dry out overnight—or perhaps even for two or three days—until it is no longer sticky. Once it's not sticky, store it in an airtight container. I'm not a huge fan of plastic generally, but I have not yet found any better kind of container for incense than heavy-duty zipper-lock freezer bags. Roll the bag around the incense, squeezing out as much air as possible. Store incense somewhere dark and cool to help preserve the scent. For long-term storage, it's best to freeze it. Everything alive dies. Everything organic decays. Incense will keep its virtues, both aesthetic and magical, for a long time, but not indefinitely. Fresh is best.

Other forms of loose incense can also be made. For example, on Mount Athos, the holy Greek mountain of the monks where women have been forbidden for more than a thousand years, cloistered monks in several of the twenty monasteries of the island produce a special type of incense, which is normally used to venerate ikons. Beginning with finely ground frankincense and aromatic woods, they add blended perfume oils to form a thick paste. The paste is kneaded by hand while chanting: "Lord Jesus Christ, Son of God, be merciful on me, a sinner." This prayer, sometimes called "the ceaseless prayer of the heart," is intoned all day long by the monks as part of their spiritual practice. The incense paste is rolled into "snakes" and cut into small pellets. Each pellet is coated in clay powder and allowed to harden for about a month.

How to Burn Loose Incense

The easiest way to use loose incense is over charcoal. You will need a metal or stoneware bowl of some type. Fill it at least an inch deep with dirt, sand, gravel, salt, or another heat sink. Plain white rice will work, but it's not ideal, because it adds a light toasty smell where the rice burns. Salt isn't always a good choice either, as it can be anathema to some spirits—including those of the dead—and also because it is not easily compostable. Sand, dirt, or rice can all be composted, along with the ashes, so that your offerings can be returned to the land.

You will also need incense charcoal, which can be purchased online or in most places that sell incense. It is generally sold in rolls of eight to twelve disks. Each disk will be fully consumed once lit, so I recommend buying them in bulk if you burn a lot of incense. Do not use barbecue charcoal, as it produces fumes that will pollute the smell of your incense and are not healthy to breathe. Charcoal can go stale; store open packages in plastic zipper-lock bags with most of the air squeezed out.

Finally, you will need tongs or a spoon to hold the charcoal while you light it and a source of fire. Because you need strong sustained fire, it's not always easy to light charcoals from a regular disposable lighter without burning your fingers. You can use a fireplace or grill lighter, or light a candle and use that flame. You can also light incense charcoal off a gas burner on a stove.* It is easiest to light charcoal by focusing the flame on an edge. Hold the edge of the charcoal directly in the flame. It will begin to spark, and the sparks should spread across the whole surface. Stale charcoal can be more difficult; light it all around the edge until the sparks spread the whole way across. Once it is lit, gently place it on your sand or other base. Most incense has a sort of bowl shape on one side. Put that side up to hold the incense.

Wait for the charcoal to glow red-hot, and then cover over with gray ash. Once the charcoal is ready, place your incense on top. One of the nice things about loose incense is that you can use however much or little you like, and you can add or change ingredients as you go. If you would like more smoke—such as for evocation—you can add a single drop of water,

---

* Use a spoon, so you don't burn yourself. I know I told you to always use a spoon, but you *really* need it if you're lighting from the stove.

which will produce an impressive but short-lasting cloud of steam, or a drop of honey, which will produce a slower, thick, heavy smoke, which is excellent for evocation or scrying.

If you would like less smoke, instead of putting the incense directly on the charcoal, here's a trick: You know the little tin cup that tea lights come in?

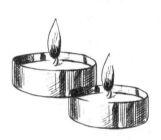

After you've burned the candle, rinse one out with hot water. It's okay if there's a little bit of wax left, but get out as much as you easily can. Put a very shallow layer of heat sink like sand or salt in the bottom of the cup, and then place the incense on top of that. Put the cup directly on top of the charcoal. This will melt and smolder the incense much more slowly, producing less smoke and extending the burn. The tins can be reused several times. You can also purchase small mica plates designed for this purpose. For magic, I often like to use a large coin, which comes out of the ritual charged as a talisman.

No matter how you use it, allow the charcoal to burn completely out and get cold before you compost it. Ideally, it should burn completely and leave nothing but ash, but that is often not the case, especially if the charcoal was stale. If you need to put incense out while it's still burning, put the whole incense bowl inside another bowl and pour water over it.

There are several other options for burning loose incense. You can use an electric burner. These are very popular in the Middle East and can be found in any Middle Eastern import shop and most halal grocers. Electric burners are a great idea if you burn a lot of incense; I have several in my home. They burn at a lower temperature, and so you get more smell but less smoke from the same amount. They're also a little more environmentally friendly, both in terms of minimizing single-use charcoal and its packaging and because they put fewer particulates into the air. They are a good option for households with people who are mildly sensitive to smoke. Every electric burner is different; read the instructions before use. Obviously, if someone is very sensitive, incense just isn't a good choice, no matter how you burn it.

Another option is to use a candle warmer, which consists of a small bowl, usually ceramic, over a tea light. Personally, I don't care for these; I find they don't really get hot enough. However, if they work for you, then that's great. Line the bowl with foil; melted resin is very difficult to clean up. You can also get an adjustable kind, where the bowl can be moved nearer and farther from the fire. Those are better, in my opinion.

You can also burn incense in a small cast-iron pan. Line it with foil and put the incense in that. Be careful; this method can produce *a lot* of smoke. I like this method when I'm processing incense around the house or need to burn large quantities of incense such as for fumigation.

Making Oils from Loose Incense

Loose incense can also be used to make magical oils. Grind the incense very fine and mix it with twice as much carrier oil. What oil you use should be determined by the purpose of the final product. Sweet almond oil is a good choice for most things, but I sometimes use olive oil, ghee, or even bear grease to add in their own magical virtues. The oil chosen will obviously impact the smell of the result. Experiment.

Once the incense is mixed into the oil, very gently warm it over a long period of time. A small slow cooker is good for this. If your slow cooker is too big, put the oil in a jar that fits inside the cooker. Fill the jar only two-thirds full and place the lid on upside down, so the jar is covered, but not sealed. Put the jar in the slow cooker and add at least three inches of water around it. Then cook it on the lowest setting for about six hours. Keep an eye on it, adding more water if required. Do not strain the oil before bottling. Instead, strain it as you use it. It will continue to infuse and get more powerful over time. If you intend to store the oil for long-term use, poke open several vitamin E capsules and add the liquid inside to the oil. Vitamin E is an antioxidant that will help prevent the oil from going rancid. However, no natural product lasts forever; fresh is always best for incense and oils. Oils store best in completely full bottles, kept in the cool dark. Air and heat are the enemies of oil preservation. For long-term storage, it's best to refrigerate or even freeze oils.

Making Baths from Incense

Most incense recipes can also be used as magical baths, although you will have to experiment with the proportions, as ingredients behave differently when brewed instead of burned. Do not grind the ingredients, but rather tie them very securely in a muslin tea bag. For most bathtubs, about two tablespoons is sufficient. In general, resins do not give up their scent very well in the bath, so it's best to leave them out. They won't hurt anything, but they're expensive, and it's better not to waste them. If you want a resin-scented bath, the easiest option is an essential oil. As with all magical baths, if you do not have a bathtub, you can brew the incense as a strong tea to pour over yourself at the end of your shower.

Making & Using Other Forms of Incense

Cones

All of the incense recipes in this book are intended to be burned loose; however, you can also grind them into a fine powder and add makko powder to make cones. Makko powder is the ground bark of the *Machilus thunbergii* tree. It is easily purchased online. While there are other options, makko powder is by far the best because it is (1) water-soluble and formable when wet, (2) smooth burning when dry, (3) mostly odorless, and (4) cheap and easy to acquire.

You'll need about one part makko powder to three parts powdered incense. Add a little bit of water to make a dough, and then form the cones. If you add too much water, just squeeze out as much as you can, and then wait for it to dry out some—or add more powder. I like to make several sizes of cones so that I can choose how much incense to burn at a time. When in doubt, err on the side of making your cones smaller rather than larger. If they're too big, they won't dry properly or burn evenly. Put the cones on wax paper and allow them to dry at room temperature. When you think they are dry, snap the biggest one in half to check. Once you are sure they are completely dry, store them in an airtight container. Include a crumpled paper towel to absorb any moisture. For long-term storage, put incense in the freezer.

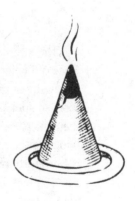

Sticks

You can also make your own incense sticks from blanks known as punks, although in my opinion it is not worth the trouble. I find incense sticks messy and wasteful. However, if you'd like to make them, grind your incense down to a very fine powder and set aside about 10 percent of it. To the rest, add close to the same amount of makko so that the resulting mixture is half makko and half incense. The exact ratio of makko you'll need is very variable, depending on the exact ingredients, their freshness, your climate, and many other factors. You'll have to experiment. Slowly add warm water until the powder comes together to form a paste. If you added too much water, add in some of the powder you reserved. Use your hands to knead the paste until it is very evenly mixed. Let it sit for several hours somewhere airtight, and remix it if it has separated. You may need to rewet it slightly. Mix the paste again.

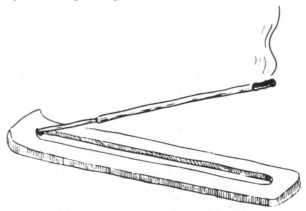

Use a bottle or rolling pin to roll it out flat, as thin as you can get it. Slice off a piece and wrap it around a blank stick. It needs to be thinner than a pencil, but the thinner you can get it, the better. It is much easier to make incense sticks by dipping them in a blend of essential oils than by rolling them in paste made from whole ingredients. Most of the recipes in this book can be adapted for use this way, but you'll need to experiment with the proportions, as essential oils differ in strength from whole components. For magical use, I strongly recommend using whole plant products, rather than essential oils, because, being closer to the living plant, they retain more of their magical character and personality.

Cigars

Incense cigars—which are sometimes improperly called smudge sticks—are another cross-culturally ubiquitous form of incense, often used for healing and purification. They can be made with any type of fresh leaf; artemisias and salvias are among the most common. Conifer needles, bark shavings, and flower petals can all be successfully incorporated, with varying degrees of difficulty. To make an incense cigar, you need to start with fresh herb cuttings. Leave the leaves attached to their stems, and spread them out to dry slightly, but not completely. You would like them to be dry, but still pliable. For most herbs, overnight will accomplish this. If they are too wet when you wrap them, they will not properly dry inside and go moldy. If they are too dry, they will be too brittle and fall apart as you wrap them.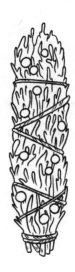

Align the cuttings to produce a cylinder the size and shape you would like. Align the tops of the cuttings, with the pieces with the thickest stems on the outside. If you have loose leaves, needles, or flowers, put them in the middle. Trim both ends even, and then carefully compress the cigar in one hand. Use the other hand to tie cotton* embroidery floss tightly around the middle. Carefully wrap down to the stem end, tie another knot, then continue wrapping up to the top. Tie another knot and wrap back down to the middle. Cut your thread and tie it off neatly. Shake the cigar so any loose pieces fall out. Allow it to dry for a few days, then examine it. You may need to add some tighter wrapping. Shake off any loose pieces, and then it's ready for use. Light one end and gently blow on it until a coal forms. Incense cigars are most often used by waving them around to suffumigate a space, but they can also be fanned or smoked like a tobacco cigar.** Incense cigars can also be rolled in cigarette papers or in cigar wrappers. This is a good choice for stealthy magic, especially if you empty a commercial cigarette and refill it with the incense of your choice.

---

*   Read the label carefully to assure it's not rayon, which stinks when burned.

**   Obviously, this is not appropriate for all plants or all people. Use appropriate caution when inhaling things.

Part Two

Ingredients

How to Use This Directory of Ingredients

IN THIS PART of the book, we'll discuss a great variety of materials you can use in your incense. However, you don't need to keep nearly that many in stock; many of the recipes in this book can be made with a pantry of just a few easy-to-acquire ingredients: a resin, an aromatic wood, an artemisia, some flower petals, and a selection of herbs and spices you can get at any grocery store. Some of the ingredients we'll discuss are difficult to ethically source. Be sure to investigate not only the farming, but also the labor, trade, and shipping practices of people from whom you buy. I've included a wide variety of ingredients for the sake of completeness, but in my own practices, I prefer to rely primarily on plants I can grow or wildcraft in my immediate environment.

Resins

AROMATIC RESINS, also called balsams, are natural plant products. While we sometimes apply the word *resin* to all sticky tree products, technically resins are not sap, but a liquid produced in special resin cells of the plant, usually in response to injury. Resins ooze out to coat wounds in the bark and then slowly solidify. While each resin is unique, they can generally be interchanged if you have a limited pantry of ingredients. All resins share a rich, woodsy smell redolent of ancient churches. If you close your eyes and conjure up the scent "incense," you are probably imagining a blend of resins. I like to imagine that the warm, delicious smell of resin incense is what wafts from heaven's bakeries.

Almost every culture on Earth uses resin as sacred incense. For example, in Europe, frankincense and myrrh are the most popular resins, which are burned in both the Catholic and Orthodox mass. This practice was imported into Europe from the Near East; neither frankincense nor myrrh will grow on that continent. In the Americas, pine and copal are the most popular and have been and still are used in a variety of ritual contexts by indigenous sacred ritualists and magicians. In Asia, dragon's blood and benzoin are used for medicinal, religious, and magical purposes.

Magically, resins are essentially solidified woodland sunshine; their sorcerous virtues are primarily solar and celestial, with an emphasis on purity, divinity, regality, and richness. They are excellent for healing, divination, and purification, as well as peace, prosperity, and love magic. Because of their history as luxury trade goods, resins are a well-received offering for most spirits and excellent for wealth, prosperity, status, and influence-drawing work. In this context, they are sometimes associated with the sphere of the planet Jupiter, although, to my mind, they are more naturally solar.

All resins have strong celestial resonance. They have a high vibration and are an excellent aid to meditation and visualization. Resin incense is also an excellent offering for all solar and sky deities and favored by most angels and celestial gods. Resins help us connect to the wisdom of the Earth and partake in communion with the trees. They are a healing balm, awakening the mind to memory, happiness, and inspiration and the soul to healing old wounds. Resins fortify the souls of the dead for their Long Journey and are an excellent offering for the Mighty and Beloved Dead.

Resin produces thick, long-lasting clouds of smoke that make an excellent medium for spirit manifestation; to promote this effect, you can add a few drops of water or honey. Additionally, many resins have mild entheogenic effects supporting clarity, openness, and tranquility. When in doubt about which sort of incense a magical operation calls for, resins are almost always a great choice! One notable exception is when working with demons, who are, generally, not fond of resins.

Wildcrafting Resin

Many of the widely known varieties of resin are dramatically overharvested and frequently raised and collected in ecologically problematic ways, often by coerced labor. Please take care in sourcing these materials. Conveniently, the most magically potent resin you can use is also the most ecologically and ethically responsible: whatever kind you can harvest in your own yard or local area. Most coniferous (evergreen, needle-bearing) trees produce some resin, although some more than others.

Get to know your own local plants. Where I live in Western Pennsylvania, eastern white pine produces the most resin and makes lovely incense. Most conifers, many deciduous (broad-leafed) trees, and some other flowering plants also produce resin, although some of those don't make great incense. I recommend collecting all resins you come across and then testing them once you get home. And it should go without saying to exercise appropriate caution when inhaling unfamiliar substances.

In order to wildcraft resin, head to wherever conifer trees grow. Take a shallow glass jar, a sturdy butter knife, and a bottle of water. The jar and the knife should be dedicated to resin work; resin is extremely difficult to clean off. You might also want rubber gloves; collecting resin can be sticky business. Look for trees with broken branches or other injuries. Examine the wound for drips of resin. Unless there are big drips and gobs, *do not* harvest. The tree needs its resin to heal; take only the excess that has dripped down. Before collecting, examine the area around the tree. Is there trash? Pick it up. Are there other things you can do for the tree? Do them.

Scrape off the excess resin and put it in the jar. Depending on how old it is, the resin may be brittle enough to break, or it might still be sticky and need to be scraped off. Resin can take a long time to dry (years). Generally, it's better to let it at least partly crystallize on the tree before harvesting, but you can also spread it thinly on wax paper and let it dry in the pantry. You can also roll balls of sticky resin in powdered herbs or other ingredients.

Whether you wildcraft or not, you may wish to powder resin. Traditionally, this is done with a mortar and pestle, but that is difficult and time-consuming. In my experience, it is well worth the investment to buy a coffee grinder dedicated to this purpose. Don't even bother trying to clean this enough to use for food again; you will never get all the resin off.

Frankincense

Frankincense, the resin of *Boswellia* trees, has a long and storied history of use throughout North Africa and the Middle East. The smell of frankincense is difficult to describe. It is warm, dry, slightly spicy, and sweet, with a scent like hot cinnamon butter prevailing. It is piney and a little lemony with a faint undertone of deep mossy woods. Higher-quality frankincense is richer and smoother, with more fruit and less acid. If you do not wildcraft your own and keep only one resin in stock, it should probably be frankincense. In what follows, I will describe the scent of other resins by comparing them to frankincense, although even different frankincenses vary from each other.

In older texts, it is often called *olibanum*, a word closely related to ancient Semitic words for "milk" and "white" and "moon." Near Eastern trade in frankincense is well documented for at least four thousand years, and most likely it is much older than that.[25] There are fifty-two references to frankincense in the Bible. Egyptian records show similarly abundant references. Frankincense trees were among the gifts brought to King Solomon by the Queen of Sheba; however, they likely withered and died since frankincense grows only in very specific climates. In fact, some ancient legends say that they will grow only in the most inhospitable of places, tended by dragons who strike out at any who attempt to gather the resin without knowing its secrets. These dragons were called the Serpents with Wings.[26]

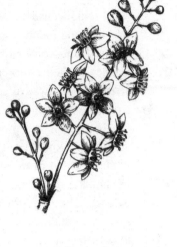

Of course, frankincense was also one of the gifts the legendary three magi brought to the infant Jesus. In some tellings of that story, frankincense is presented by the mage Melchior from Arabia. His name means "King of Light," and he blesses the infant Christ as the incarnation of the Divine Light, just as frankincense is a physical embodiment of the sun's light.

Although extremely pleasant to us humans, the scent of frankincense repulses many flying insects; it has long been used as a mosquito repellent in the Middle East and North Africa.[27] It is perhaps this that led to its reputation as a magical pest repellent as well. Few unpleasant spirits or energies can easily withstand fumigation with frankincense. To use it for this purpose, close all the doors and windows in the room, and take the batteries out of the smoke detector. Burn *a lot* of frankincense; hot box the entire room with the smoke. This is also an effective treatment for sickrooms. For prophylactic spiritual cleansing, it can be burned in more manageable amounts while carrying it counterclockwise around the room. Whenever you banish unwanted spirits and energies, you should end by inviting in wanted ones. Nature abhors a vacuum.

Frankincense has been shown to have an uplifting effect on the emotions and guard against anxiety.[28] Recent research indicates it may be a mild hallucinogen, a fact long attested to. For example, in the Babylonian Talmud,[29] we are told that a prisoner slated for execution was given wine in which frankincense had been dissolved, in order to "confuse his mind and thereby minimize his suffering." In Jordan, frankincense is considered an aphrodisiac and thought to promote virility and fertility. Magically, frankincense promotes courage, joy, success, and pure love.

Frankincense is used in Traditional Chinese Medicine to improve learning and memory, especially in the elderly. It is also traditionally used by pregnant women to ensure a powerful memory and exceptional intelligence in their children. In the West, frankincense is reputed to open the senses, both physical and spiritual. Although it is very safe, please consult a doctor or qualified herbalist before taking frankincense as medicine.

In my personal practice, the ur-spirit Frankincense most often appears as a black-skinned old man, richly dressed in cloth of gold. He has long white hair and beard and wears an elaborate fez of yellow, red, and gold. He holds a dark wood box chased with gold. It is full of glowing frankincense. These anthropomorphisms are very personal; that is not the true form of Frankincense, but a form he takes for me. Yours might very well look different.

Myrrh

Myrrh, the resin of several species of *Commiphora* trees, has a long history as a funeral incense and also in more hands-on work with the dead. It was used in ancient Egypt as part of the embalming process and continued to be a standard feature of European funerals until the 15th century.

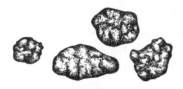

A fifth-dynasty mural from Egypt depicts the king Sahure tending a myrrh tree and bears the inscription "Sahure's splendor soars up to heaven."[30] Like frankincense, with which it is often paired, myrrh has a rich biblical history, which associates it strongly with Queen Esther, and thus with the goddess Ishtar. It was a key ingredient in ketoret, the sacred temple incense of ancient Israel.* In ancient Greece, Myrrha was a girl transformed into a myrrh tree by Aphrodite after her father impregnated her, accused her of seducing him, and then tried to kill her. The infant she gave birth to—in tree form—is immortal Adonis, for whom women weep. The tears of all mortal women mix with those of his mother—shining golden tears of myrrh. In Christian myth, myrrh (like frankincense) is a gift of the magi to the infant Jesus. Most often, myrrh is the offering of Balthazar, a young mage of color from Yemen. Just as

---

* See the ketoret recipe in the final chapter of this book.

frankincense represents Jesus's divinity, myrrh symbolizes his mortality and the power of his death.

There are those who believe that our modern myrrh is not the same as that referred to by the ancients, but to my knowledge, there is little direct evidence of this. Researchers at the University of Florence have discovered that myrrh acts on opioid receptors in the brain—at least in mice.[31] Myrrh is darker, heavier, muskier, nuttier, and more medicinal smelling than frankincense. Good myrrh has a stanky biological smell at the bottom, which can tend toward licorice in cheaper varieties.

In addition to the solar and arboreal qualities all resins share, myrrh's magical uses tend toward the saturnine and lunar. It also has strong Underworld resonance; it is an excellent offering for the dead and for most chthonic deities. In the same vein, it is a powerful aid for magic designed to heal grief, release mortality fear, and address past-life issues.

Medicinally, myrrh is used primarily as an antiseptic, and its magical character has this flavor as well. Myrrh is excellent to combat the miasma of a sickroom. For coughs and colds, oil added to a humidifier is often preferable to incense smoke.

Myrrh can also be directly addressed as a spirit ally, as in this spell from Greco-Egyptian late antiquity, which I have interpreted in English. In the papyrus, it is used as a coercive love spell, but the final line explains that it can be for all purposes as a frame around a petition. You will need both a long and short form of the petition.

A PETITION SPELL TO BE SAID OVER MYRRH

BASED ON GREEK MAGICAL PAPYRUS[32] IV 1496–1595

Myrrh, antidote, severe one of the flames,

Intercessor, reconciler, you who sets spirits ablaze.

Myrrh is your name among the profane

But I call to you now by your secret names:

I call Sarcophagus, Flesh-eater, the Scorcher of Hearts.

I call on you now, and charge you to depart,

Not to distant Araby, nor far Babylon,

But only to work my will as a goodwill liaison:

    [insert full petition here]

Do all this because I adjure you by the three holy names:
ANUXO ABRASAX TRO
And by your stronger and more forceful names:
KORMEIOTH IAŌ SABAOTH ADONAI.
Bring my request to completion, oh, Myrrh.
As you lend your potency to the flames,

    [short-form petition goes here]

I who am NAME, whose mother is NAME,
I beseech you by the secret names:
MARPARKOURITH NASAARI
NAIEMARE PAIPARI NEKOURI.
I throw you into the burning flames,
And I beseech you by the immortal and almighty god.
I beseech you again:
ADONAI BARBAR IAŌ ZAGOURE
HARSAMOSI ALAOUS & SALAOS.

I beseech you who uphold human lives.
Listen, Listen, oh, Great God:
ADONAI ETHYIA.
Self-begetting and everlasting god
EIOE IAŌ AIŌ
PHNEOS SPHINTES ARBATHIAŌ
IAŌ IAE IŌA AI.

You who are

OUER GONTHALOR RARAEL

ABRA BRACHA

SOROORMEROHEGAR MARBAPHRIOROGX

IAŌ SABAOTH

MASKELLI MASKELLO

AMONSOE ANOCH RIGX PHNOUKENTABAOTH

SOUSAE OHINPHESECH MAPHI RAR

ANOURIN IBANOTH AROUER CHNOUPH

ANOCH BATHI OUCH IARBAS

BABAUBAR ELOAI.

    [insert short-form petition here]

Do it now, in this day, in this night, in this very hour!
MOULOTH
PHOPHITH PHTHOITH PHTHOYTH PENON.
I call on you also, who hold the power,
PHTHAN ANOCH,

Give heed to me, only-begotten one,
MANEBIA BAI CHYRIRUOTH
THADEIN ADONAI EROU NOUNI
MIOONX XOUTIAI MARMARAUOTH.

    [short-form petition]

Now, Now, Now!

Immediately, Immediately!

Quick! Quick! Quick!

Pine

Eastern white pine (*Pinus strobus*) is called "Tree of Peace" by the Haudenosaunee (Iroquois) people. This title derives from its pivotal role in the creation of the Great Peace (Kayanerenh-kowa). It is native to the northeastern United States and parts of southeastern Canada. White pine is the resin I most often wildcraft. In the western United States, piñon pine predominates. I have very little experience with living piñon, but its resin is difficult to distinguish from that of white pine. In my opinion, unless you are specifically awakening them as representatives of a particular ecoregion or using them in the context of traditional Native practices, all pine resins are interchangeable.

Because they are inexpensive, hardy, and low maintenance, pines are often planted in public parks, graveyards, and other public spaces, which are all excellent places to collect resin. As you might expect, resin collected in graveyards is especially good for working with the dead. Here in Western Pennsylvania, and through the Northeast, white pines are often used as Christmas trees. If you ask nicely when they are not busy, many Christmas tree lots will allow you to collect resin from their trees.

Pine resin is a surely a scent you'll recognize from pine-scented cleaners, which are historically made from pine tar. It is sharp, clean, and slightly citrusy. Pine is antiseptic and cleansing, and its magical uses follow suit. It is excellent for purification and healing work and lends clarity to psychic vision. It is good to draw things out, particularly spiritual infections and psychic intrusions. For this use, it is sometimes blended with camphor. Pine needles are also excellent for incense; collect them along with the resin. Among the Haudenosaunee, the needles are burned in spring and fall, filling the home with cleansing smoke.

In addition to her importance as a magical ally, White Pine is also a great survival ally. Pine needle tea is high in vitamin C and excellent for warding off illness. The inner cambium is also edible, but not delicious. The resin can be used to waterproof and seal things, from canoes to small wounds.

For most readers of this book, pine is likely to be the only famous resin tree that grows in your area. It is well worth your time to acquaint yourself with this tree, not just as a source of materials, but as a spiritual ally in its own right.

Chios Mastic

Chios mastic, the resin of *Pistacia lentiscus*, is a less common resin that is close to my heart. It is native only to the Greek island of Chios, off the western shore of Turkey, and harvested in twenty-four small "mastic villages," which have been the sole caretakers of the trees since the Byzantine Era. My family legend tells that my great-grandmother Katherine's family survived the Chios massacre of 1822 only because they tended the trees and the sultan wished to have mastiha for his court. The taste and smell of Chios mastic are similar to copal, but with a slightly lighter, sunnier, younger smell. It can have notes of licorice or almonds.

Many of my older relatives used to chew mastic like gum; they say it settles the stomach. This tradition is very old—Hippocrates recommends chewing mastic as a breath freshener. In fact, the word *mastic* is closely related to the Greek word for chewing, and the English word *masticate*.

In antiquity, mastic was imported into Egypt, where it was used as incense, medicine, a spice for food, and also in embalming. It is a key ingredient in the Egyptian incense called kyphi, which we'll discuss further in the final chapter of the book. Magically, Chios mastic is even more solar than frankincense and has a slightly more oceanic feel. It is excellent for clarity and purification; it is often a key ingredient in chrism (Christian holy oil). Chios mastic is also a magical material par excellence for glamour magic and spells to attract romantic partners.

Copal

Copal is a name given to resins from many different kinds of trees native to South and Central America. Many of the cultures of pre-Columbian Mesoamerica burned copal ceremonially without distinguishing between sources. When purchased commercially in the United States, copal is most often *Protium copal*.

The English word *copal* is derived from the Nahuatl word *copalli*, which means "incense," and copal resins have a long history of use across many peoples in Central and South America. Today, copal is used by indigenous peoples in southern Mexico and Central America during sweat lodge ceremonies as well as sacred mushroom ceremonies.

Like all resins, copal is excellent for purification, banishing, and healing. It is an excellent all-around temple incense. The smell of most copal is lighter than frankincense, similar to Chios mastic, but less fruity.

Dragon's Blood

Dragon's blood is a colloquial name applied to a wide variety of bright red resins. When purchased commercially, it is most often from a genus of rattan palm called *Daemonorops*. In the ancient Mediterranean, the most common type was *Dracaena cinnabari*. Owing to its color and association with dragons, dragon's blood is somewhat more martial than other resins. In addition to its use in incense, dragon's blood resin is often ground and applied to color varnish, paint, dye, or ink. Dragon's blood has almost no smell raw and a mildly fruity, sweet, and only slightly resinous smell when burned.

As incense or ink, dragon's blood is excellent for aggressive magic, as well as that involving defense from aggression. For a quick protective ward, walk smoking dragon's blood around the boundaries of your home, clockwise, three times. Leave piles of dragon's blood in each corner. Because of its association with blood, it is also potent magic for both the physical and metaphoric heart.

The ancient Greek name for dragon's blood tree, *drakaina*, means "she-dragon" and is also a magical name for several goddesses, including Hekate, Athena, and Demeter. In my work, I often call upon Great Drakaina, an Underworld avatar of Hekate who teaches oracular prophecy and shape-shifting. Dragon's blood is an excellent aid in draconic shape-shifting work. To use it for this purpose, huff the smoke and practice imagining you are breathing fire.

Aromatic Woods

MOST WOODS smell pleasant when burned, from pine's nostalgic campfire scent through the barbecue tang of hickory, from sandalwood's creaminess to the medicinal smell of camphor. Whenever you have access to sawdust, wood chips, or twigs, I recommend burning them to see what they'll be like as incense. However, beware of commercial lumber, which is sometimes treated with nasty chemicals you don't want to breathe. When you're in the woods, sniff all the trees! If one smells good, it will probably smell even better burning. Gather all sorts of leaves and needles, along with small twigs, and experiment with them at home. If you don't know what kind of tree you're gathering from, make sure to take photos, so you can get someone else to identify it. Obviously, some degree of caution needs to be exercised when experimenting with breathing unfamiliar things. Experiment outside, and burn only a small twig, *not* powdered wood. Twigs burn slowly enough that even if you're burning poisonous wood, you will not inhale enough to hurt you. A few trees I recommend against burning are yew, which is poisonous in large quantities, and ailanthus, or tree of heaven, an invasive plant that smells *very bad* when burned.

Sandalwood

Sandalwood is harvested from several parasitic plants of the genus *Santalum*. It is legendary as an incense, particularly in India and the Far East. Its fame among aromatic woods owes primarily to the fact that its fragrance is very shelf-stable, even when ground. Sadly, this has led to it being overharvested; take care when sourcing sandalwood. White, or Indian, sandalwood (*Santalum album*) is a vulnerable species; I do not recommend its use. Red,

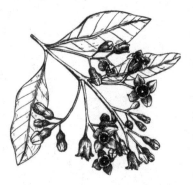

or Australian, sandalwood (*Santalum spicatum*) is commercially cultivated in—you guessed it!—Australia and a better choice, although still not as good as your own native aromatic woods. White sandalwood is beginning to be grown in Australia as well, but the trees take a long time to mature, and it is not widely available for harvest yet.

The scent of sandalwood is difficult to describe, but familiar to most people as "oriental incense." It is creamy, rich, delicate, and warm. It smells like I imagine fairy breast milk would. It is very common in Hindu religious practice; its Sanskrit name is *chandana*. Sandalwood is especially sacred to Shiva and Lakshmi. It is sometimes ground and mixed with water to make a paste, which is used for anointing idols, worshippers, and ritual items. Sometimes, saffron is added to this paste.

Like all luxury trade goods, sandalwood denotes richness and is excellent in wealth-drawing work. It also improves focus during meditation and trance. Like most plants that figured into Egyptian mummification practices, it makes an excellent offering for the Mighty Dead—although I prefer cedar for that. In Korean spirit work, it serves as a World Tree, or Tree of Life. It is an excellent offering for most divine spirits, as an accompaniment to prayer. The angel Sandalphon, whose name is etymologically unrelated to sandalwood, but who has become associated with it in folklore, is said to gather the incense and prayers of all people and weave them into wreaths to crown G-d's head. In modern Anglophone paganism, sandalwood is often used for purification and healing; both are within the scope of its traditional use. Because of its parasitic nature, sandalwood is also excellent in bane work, but be sure to specifically awaken its parasitism for such use.

Cedar

Technically, *cedar* refers only to trees of the genus *Cedrus*, native to the Himalayas and the mountains of the Mediterranean. Perhaps the most famous of these are the legendary cedars of Lebanon, *Cedrus libani*. However, in American English, the name applies to a much wider variety of aromatic trees, including California incense cedar (*Calocedrus decurrens*), western red cedar (*Thuja plicata*), and white cedar, also called eastern arborvitae (*Thuja occidentalis*). *Juniperus virginiana* is sometimes called eastern red cedar, but it's more properly a juniper, so I'll talk about it with them below. Cedar is among the most common incense plants in North America, used by both native and immigrant magicians and spirit workers. The wood and needles can be used in incense interchangeably.

All cedars are excellent offerings for celestial spirits and for the dead. For example, cedar of Lebanon was the wood of choice for coffins in ancient Egypt. When Osiris was killed by Set and his coffin set adrift, it found its final resting place in a cedar tree. Like many magical and practical uses of cedar, its employment for coffins is underlain by its rot and insect resistance, which lend it an air of immortality. This insect resistance also leads to its use in a variety of containers, from small boxes to large chests and even walk-in closets. When I was young, the house where we lived had a cedar closet, which was attached to my bedroom. As a teenager, I used it as my magical working temple, and the smell of cedar is still intimately tied up in my magic.

My local cedar is mostly arborvitae, or white cedar. It's native in the colder parts of my ecoregion and common everywhere in the Northeast. Because it grows tall, straight, and fast, it makes an excellent wind and privacy screen and is frequently used in commercial landscaping. White Cedar is a wonderful ally for both magic and survival, and one with a deep and sacred past. Her Anishinaabe name is Nookomis Giizhik, or Grandmother Cedar; she holds the north in their medicine wheel.[33]

Magically, cedar is most often used as a World Tree, as well as a purifier and protector. Like many purifying plants, cedar can also be used as an abortifacient, but I do not recommend it for this purpose. The Anishinaabe hang cedar wreaths on their doors to protect from unwelcome visitors and above their beds to prevent bad dreams. In modern powwow, the audience is asperged with a cedar bough before some dances. The mouth is washed out with cedar needle tea after meals, and this practice has a magical cleansing action as well. Cedar is a remarkable air freshener;

place boughs in sickrooms and other places that need a serious reboot. In oil form, it is common in sweat lodge ceremonies. Among the Haudenosaunee, hunters bathe in cedar-scented steam before they set out.[34] The Chippewa burn fresh twigs during ritual.[35]

Legend says that cedar trees are perfectly symmetrical; that their crown and roots are just the same shape. One story tells that if a mother bird built a nest on a certain branch, a mother rabbit would surely dig a burrow below the corresponding root. Cedar unites the worlds and incarnates the cosmic balance. As an incense, cedar carries our prayers and spells up the heavens *and* down into the underworld. This is part of Cedar's function as a World Tree. Cedar incense is an excellent choice for journey work.

Cedar is an outstanding addition to incenses that need an uplifting element. It is also good for working with the dead, especially beloved ancestors. It opens the psychic senses, and—more importantly—it opens the mind to messages we might not otherwise consider. However, cedar can also be used to cast out. Cedar is a tree of insight. Among the Potawatomi, cedar needles are burned on coals as part of exorcism rites and to purify sacred objects,[36] and I use it for that purpose as well.

Cypress & Juniper

Cypress is a common name for many different trees of the family Cupressaceae. The name derives* from the Greek Kyparissos, a young man of Chios who became the lover of Apollo—or sometimes Sylvanus—and was eventually transformed into the cypress tree. Cypress is closely associated with mourning and the underworld; it is an excellent offering for the Beloved Dead. Among the cypresses are the junipers, which are often used in Siberian and Russian magical incenses.

Mediterranean cypress, also called Tuscan cypress, is beloved as an ornamental tree and has been cultivated for millennia. The trees themselves can grow to be very, very old. Because of this reputation for immortality, they were used extensively as offerings for the dead. In ancient Greece, juniper was sacred to the Furies and often burned as an offering to the infernal gods. It was woven into wreaths for Pluto, and Athenian houses in

---

* Although there is a long tradition of providing etymologies for plant names based in mythology, in fact the myths almost certainly arise later to describe the plant.

mourning were decked with boughs of cypress. It was used extensively in Roman funeral rites, including being placed on cremation pyres. Among the ancient Hebrews it was also a sign of mourning and remains a popular decorative element on Israeli gravestones.

Where I live, and throughout much of the eastern United States, the most common native cypress is eastern juniper (*Juniperus virginiana*), also called eastern red cedar, although it is not, technically, a cedar. It is a very long-lived tree—one in West Virginia is 940 years old—and this adds to its reputation for wisdom and invulnerability. A pioneer species, it appears quickly in areas disturbed by wildfire or human devastation, like construction sites. The wood is highly rot resistant, and so it is often used for fence posts. It has been employed in this way since American prehistory and continues to serve in modern construction. This association with boundaries and crossroads makes it an excellent magical material in the sphere of Mercury.

Junipers generally, and eastern red cedar in particular, are an excellent aid to trance. Like most witching plants, it is an abortifacient in large doses, and it has historically been used among the Cherokee for this purpose.[37] Like all cypresses, eastern red cedar has a strong underworld connection and is very appropriate in incense offered to the dead. It is burned among the Lakota at funerals and left on grave sites among the Chippewa.[38]

Like all cypresses, eastern red cedar is also a powerful ally for protection. It grows strong, straight, and tall, standing like a warrior. Among the Navajo, eastern red cedar is the wood of choice for the wands carried during the War Dance,[39] and it is used by the Dakota to make lightning rods.[40] eastern red cedar does not keep away trouble; it faces it head-on. It is not a good choice in long-acting protection work, such as all-purpose warding. Rather, call on cypress to protect you when all other options have failed and you are about to walk into danger.

Cherry & Other Fruit Woods

My favorite aromatic wood to burn is cherry. When I was little, we had an old ornamental Japanese cherry tree in our yard who was my beloved friend and my first incarnate World Tree. His pink blossoms rained down like Seussical snow just as school let out for the summer. That floral confetti was the most magical thing I could imagine. On the rare occasions we built a fire in our fireplace, my father always included some cherrywood for its delightful smell. Although I personally adore Japanese cherry (*Prunus serrulata*) for nostalgic reasons, wild or black cherry (*Prunus serotina*) is even better as an incense and native to most of the eastern United States. The bark is also excellent in incense and highly medicinal.

Cherrywood has a sweet fruity woodsy/herbal smell, with an occasional hint of vanilla. Many people smoke or grill meat with cherrywood to impart its taste to the meat. For the most part, all fruit woods are interchangeably magically; I just happen to have a personal relationship with cherry. Cherry and other fruit woods are excellent for divination and purification, and particularly good for love and fertility magic. During divination, it clears the mind and opens the heart. It is a favored offering of the Fair Folk and also good for most spirits of the spheres of Venus or the Moon.

All parts of the cherry tree are excellent for sex and love magic. Feed a beloved enchanted cherry pie made with cherry fruit, vanilla, cinnamon, and brown sugar to ensure their lust for you. Carry a cherry pit in your left pocket to find a new lover, or place one under a pillow to dream of your intended. Burn cherry incense under a spring full moon to learn to love yourself. Meditate under a blossoming cherry tree to seek audience with Aphrodite to ask her to shower you with her blessings. To help a woman conceive, prepare a paste of native soil and cherry juice, and paint a spiral, clockwise out from her naval, on her belly before sex.

Camphor

Traditionally, camphor is distilled from the wood of the ho tree, which is also called camphor laurel (*Cinnamomum camphora*), an Asian tree naturalized—and sometimes invasive—in the southern United States. It is perhaps a little bit of a cheat to place it in this chapter, as we usually do not burn the wood itself, but the pure chemical $C_{10}H_{16}O$, which, today, is usually distilled from turpentine. Camphor is a powerful purifier and protectant. It was used as a fumigant to ward off the Black Death and many other plagues and is a less toxic alternative to mothballs. It is both antimicrobial and insecticidal. Like most materials with those properties, it is just as effective against incorporeal parasites and pests. It can be burned alone for purification and cleansing, although I prefer to mix it with mugwort for this purpose.

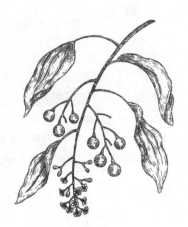

Camphor is an excellent offering to lunar spirits and good to promote clarity in divination, oneiromancy, and trance work. To prevent nightmares, put a piece of camphor in a glass of water, and set it near the bedside. Camphor smoke itself can be used for divination. Ask a yes/no question directly to the incense, exhorting it to speak truely, as it always does. If the smoke rises in a straight column, the answer is yes, but if it wavers and leans, the answer is no. There are further details on incense divination at the beginning of the spellwork chapter.

The ho tree, and camphor in particular, is sacred to the Egyptian goddess Het-heru (Hathor) and was often used in Egyptian perfumes and love spells. Camphor is also common in Romany love spells, which were sometimes called "Gypsy" or "Egyptish" in old books, leading to some confusion between the two. On the other hand, camphor is also used to shake off an ex-lover or break couples up, often in conjunction with pennyroyal.

In Guernsey, camphor was used as an apotropaic charm to ward off malicious witchcraft. For this application, place camphor, salt, and heather in a white linen bag and wear on a ribbon around the neck so that the sachet rests above the heart. Another similar charm is slightly more complicated:

> Take nine bits of green broom, and two sprigs of the same, which you must tie together in the form of a cross; nine morsels of elder, nine leaves of betony, nine of agrimony, a little bay salt, salammoniac [sic], new wax, barley, leaven, camphor, and quick-silver. The quick-silver must be inclosed in cobbler's wax. Put the whole into a new linen cloth which has never been used, and sew it well up so that nothing may fall out. Hang this round your neck. It is a sure preservative against the power of the witches.[41]

Place squares of camphor in the corners of a room to ward and protect it from malicious spirits, malefic magic, and spiritual impurity. It can also be burned as incense and walked clockwise around the perimeter of a space three times for this purpose. Asperging with rosemary is a good addition to this.

Myrtle

Myrtle (*Myrtus communis*, or other species of *Myrtus*) is a common garden plant in warm climates. It cannot overwinter where I live, so I have no experience with the living plant. It is native to the Mediterranean and has a

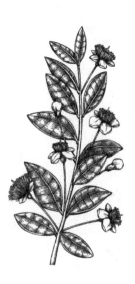

long history of use in religion and magic and is still extensively used in Jewish ritual, particularly as part of a wand called a *lulav*.* It has a clean, slightly medicinal, mildly floral scent and taste. You've probably eaten it, even if you didn't know it. You know the weird "peppercorns" in fancy baloney? Those aren't peppercorns, they're myrtle berries. Both twigs and leaves can be burned as incense, as well as the flower and berries.

Myrtles are closely associated with the Great Goddess in her many forms. In Greece, myrtle was sacred to both Aphrodite and Demeter, and in Rome to Venus. Myrtles were planted in Aphrodite's temple gardens, and she is often depicted with myrtle wreaths. A hero's crown of myrtle signified a victory won without bloodshed, and myrtle crowns were also worn by both brides and grooms being married. In Hebrew, myrtle is called Hadassah, which is another name for the biblical queen, herself a shadow of Ishtar, to whom myrtle is especially sacred.

Myrtle is a symbol of peace, paradise, and loving marriage. Since featuring prominently in the marriage of Queen Victoria, myrtle has bedecked all British royal brides. In modern paganism, myrtle is associated with Beltane. Magically, myrtle promotes deep and lasting love and helps bring comfort and hope to those who despair. It is especially good for working through regret.

---

* *Lulav* is actually a name for a date palm frond, which is bound with boughs of myrtle and willow to make a wand.

Palo Santo

Palo santo (*Bursera graveolens* or *Bulnesia sarmienti*) is a critically over-harvested plant native to South and Central America, closely related to frankincense. It has a long history of use as a purifying incense in indigenous cultures of its native region. Traditionally, only fallen branches are harvested, and this is the only legal way to harvest it in Peru. However, its increasing popularity among nonindigenous people has led to significant poaching. Regulated, commercial cultivation has begun, but most of those trees are not yet big enough for harvesting. For these reasons, I do not recommend palo santo for people who are not working in its native context. If you choose to use it, please be cautious with your sourcing. In my limited experience, its purifying action can be replicated with most aromatic woods or resins, particularly cedar. To substitute for the scent, mix frankincense with a small amount of dried apple and a tiny bit of black pepper. This will not produce a scent masquerading as palo santo, the way a synthetic does, but rather a scent with similar qualities, which can be used in similar ways.

Agarwood

Agarwood or oud, also called aloeswood, refers to heartwood trees of the genus *Aquilaria* (lign aloes) when infected with the fungus *Phialophora parasitica*. The infection causes the tree to secrete a special type of resin (agar), which infuses the heartwood of the tree. The smell of agarwood is rich and complex, partaking of perfume scents and sweet florals, with creamy and sexually primal elements. If you imagine the scent of the magic of *One Thousand and One Nights*, the smell you're imagining is oud. Agarwood is extremely expensive and critically overharvested. However, it has recently started to be cultivated instead of wildcrafted, which will hopefully take some pressure off as the industry expands. Experts say that a significant amount of commercial agarwood is fake. Because of this, and because it is so expensive and

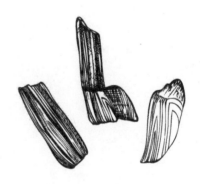

difficult to source ethically, I do not work with agarwood, and I do not recommend you do either.

Thunderstruck Oak

Wood from oak trees that have been struck by lightning is especially potent in a wide variety of magic. In incense, oak—thunderstruck or not—smells like you expect burning wood to smell: cozy as a hearth and primal as a bonfire. Although its smell is not especially lovely, I often include it in magic where I want to call upon the power of lightning—useful for bane work as well as illumination—or as an offering for spirits of the sphere of Jupiter. If you find thunderstruck oak, I recommend collecting as much wood as you can for magical use. In addition to the small amount you might use in incense, larger pieces of thunderstruck oak make wands and staves of great power, and small pieces are an excellent choice for crafting both divinatory rune sets and magical rune staves.

Herbs

Almost all herbs can be used in incense; I encourage you to experiment with whatever you have in your kitchen and whatever grows in your immediate area. Below, I discuss just a few of my favorites.

Artemisia

Artemisia is a large genus of herbs, the most important of which in incense making are mugwort, wormwood, sagebrush, and tarragon. Nearly all artemisia can be used in incense. As the name implies, all of these plants are closely associated with Artemis and with the Moon. Most artemisia are extremely bitter-tasting, but only a few have an unpleasant smell. The ubiquity of artemisia as a witching herb cannot be overstated; everywhere that it grows, it is beloved of healers, spirit speakers, and sorcerers.

MUGWORT

Mugwort, *Artemisia vulgaris*, is an extremely powerful plant ally, renowned for its ability to open the inner senses and aid in spirit flight. Although it is not native to the United States, it has naturalized in most of North America. Where I live in Pittsburgh, it is ubiquitous. I find it growing in abandoned lots and roadside ditches all the time. If you gather it wild, the best time to do so is before the flowers bloom. Here in Pittsburgh, that usually happens in August. Be careful about planting mugwort; it can be very invasive and difficult to contain.

The ancient poem called "Wodan's Nine Herbs Charm" says of it: "Remember, Mugwort, what you revealed, what you established at the

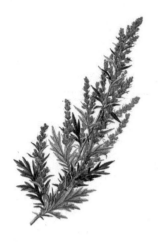

mighty proclamation: 'Una' you are called, oldest of herbs. You may avail against 3 and against 30; you may avail against poison and against contagion; you may avail against the loathsome one who travels through the land."[42]

In Traditional Chinese Medicine, mugwort cigars are burned close to acupuncture points in a process called moxibustion in English. Moxibustion is used to treat a wide variety of disorders, often in conjunction with acupuncture. Inhalation of mugwort smoke has been clinically proven to slow the heartbeat and calm the nervous system.[43] It is also used as a digestive tonic and to treat headaches. It can be applied medicinally to bring on a late period, to ease menstrual cramps, or to help increase fetal movement in breech pregnancies. Mugwort is also sometimes used as an abortifacient, but it's not very effective for this purpose. However, like all abortifacients, it is sacred to the Witch Queens.

Roman soldiers are said to have worn sprigs of mugwort in their boots to soothe sore feet and prevent fatigue. It is also excellent in the bath to ease sore feet and legs. When gathered for these purposes, it is tradition to collect it by night, while reciting "*Tollam te Artemisia ne lassus in via*" ("I take of you, Artemisia, lest I grow weary on the road"). Modern herbalists often use mugwort against athlete's foot, and it is a common ingredient in herbal shoe liners.

Among several Native American peoples, mugwort is used to calm the restless dead. For example, among the Miwok, it is extensively used in the funeral ritual and worn by mourners while sleeping to prevent unwanted visitation from the dead.[44]

In incense, mugwort smells woodsy, green, and herbal. It is one of my favorite bases for incense because, when ground, it produces a sort of fluff into which other ingredients mix well. Mugwort incense is a very effective insect repellent, and it is just as effective against spiritual pests. For example, the Schola Medica Salernitana (the Medical School of Salerno), the most important early medieval medical school in Europe, taught that mugwort "combats bad thoughts, and the devil flees from the plant."[45] Folklore teaches us that mugwort keeps away the evil eye and protects from many kinds of bane work. To promote cleansing and banishing, mugwort is often woven into the bristles of witch's besoms and brooms. Mugwort can be burned on its own for a powerful purification and banishing incense. It burns well in cigar form, and you can also buy premade moxa cigars online or at most Chinese herbalists.

Maud Grieve says in *A Modern Herbal*: "In the Middle Ages, the plant was known as Cingulum Sancti Johannis [the belt of Saint John], as it is believed that John the Baptist wore a girdle of it in the wilderness . . . a crown made from its sprays was worn on St. John's Eve to gain security from evil possession, and in Holland and Germany one of its names is St. John's Plant, because of the belief that, if gathered on St. John's Eve, it gave protection against diseases and misfortunes."[46]

Mugwort is excellent in all sorts of magic related to dreaming, journeying, and divination. Many people stuff dream pillows full of mugwort or hang a bundle over their bed to help prevent nightmares and promote lucid dreaming. However, be cautious about this; mugwort is closely related to ragweed, and many people are allergic to its pollen. That is rarely a problem in incense, because the pollen literally burns away, but exercise appropriate caution with highly allergic people. In addition to being used as an incense to promote dreaming and psychism, mugwort can be smoked from a pipe for a more powerful effect. Many people brew it as a tea; personally, I find the taste intolerably gross. Washing crystal balls and scrying mirrors with mugwort tea to promote clarity and insight is common in modern Wicca and also among non-Wiccan witches.

WORMWOOD

Wormwood (*Artemisia absinthium*) grows in similar regions as mugwort. In fact, they are so similar that they can be difficult to tell apart. Wormwood leaves are slightly more silver and rounded, and it usually has yellow flowers instead of pink. As the name implies, wormwood is an excellent treatment for parasitic worm infections in humans or animals. It can be applied directly to the skin to help soothe and heal bugbites. Wormwood can also be used to treat fever, headache, depression, and memory loss. It is also fabled as an aphrodisiac and a source of poetic and artistic inspiration. However, it is most famous as a bitter flavoring in alcohol. Several types of beer are flavored with wormwood, as are vermouth and wormwood's Latin namesake, absinthe.

Wormwood is a very mild hallucinogen, particularly in alcohol. This effect is slight in incense, unless you huff quite a lot of it. In incense, wormwood can generally be used in place of mugwort except that it is not very good for banishing. In fact, wormwood is among the best summoning incenses. Traditionally, it is burned in cemeteries to seek necromantic oracles; the spirits appear in the smoke. More instructions for using incense as a medium of spirit manifestation can be found with the Ooky Spooky Evocation Smoke in the section on divination. Like mugwort, wormwood is excellent for inducing trance, for divination or any other purpose. It is particularly good for work with the dead and the Fair Folk. It can also be used to induce the swoon of love. It is not especially pleasant-smelling when burned.

SAGEBRUSH

Sagebrush or blue sage (*Artemisia tridentata*) is the artemisia most common in the western United States, although several other related species are also called sagebrush. The Lakota name for sagebrush means "big gray bush," and sagebrush is indeed a lovely silvery color, which gives the western plains their color. Sagebrush is not a sage; it is an artemisia, closely related to mugwort. Because it does not grow near me, I don't know as much about sagebrush, but my experience has been that all artemisia are more or less interchangeable for most magical purposes.

Like its native habitat, sagebrush is hotter and drier than mugwort. Compared to mugwort, sagebrush is slightly more straightforward and aggressive, while mugwort is sneakier and more seductive. It is burned for purification and smudging, as well as being used to treat a variety of medical conditions, including headaches and colds. The Zuni Pueblo people use sagebrush to treat the foot in much the same way mugwort is used.[47] Among the Paiute, dancers asperse themselves with sagebrush boughs to purify themselves.[48] The Gosiute of Utah consider it a panacea, good for all ills.[49]

TARRAGON

Tarragon (*Artemisia dracunculus*) grows wild in many parts of North America and is also widely cultivated in gardens. The English name *tarragon* comes from the Arabic word *tarkun*, or "dragon," and the Latin name also references those creatures. Some say this is because tarragon's roots curl like dragon tails, but others say it is because it is proof positive against their venom.

Most domesticated tarragon cannot reproduce by seed; however, it spreads quickly by rhizomes. Tarragon is the most delicious of the artemisia, far less bitter than its sisters. Americans are most often familiar with its taste from béarnaise sauce, but in Eastern Europe it is used to flavor bright green soda. Both wild and domesticated tarragon can be substituted for other artemisia in most incense recipes. You should use less, because the scent of tarragon is stronger than other artemisia. Compared with other artemisia, tarragon is slightly more fiery, which makes it excellent in martial or protective work, particularly when that work would benefit from an alliance with draconic spirits. Tarragon is helpful for courage and strength before going into battle—literally or metaphorically—although in most contexts, I prefer thyme for this. Tarragon can also be used in love magic. For example, it is a common ingredient in Omaha love spells.[50] Personally, I rarely use tarragon in this way.

Lamiaceae

The Lamiaceae are a huge family of related herbs, varieties of which are found all over the world, particularly in the Northern Hemisphere. Many familiar herbs are members of this family, including most of those in this chapter.

MINT

Mints, the large genus *Mentha*, are the most common members of the Lamiaceae family, which is sometimes called the mint family. Because mints very easily hybridize, expect interesting results if you plant multiple mints together. Mint is extremely easy to grow in any moist environment. It's best to grow mint in a container; it can spread invasively.

Most mints can easily be identified by their familiar smell. Like most strongly smelling plants, it is good against pests, both literal and figurative. Mints' smell is due to the chemical menthol ($C_{10}H_{20}O$), which is used in a wide variety of applications from cigarettes to medicine. This is what produces the cooling sensation common to mints, as well as their analgesic properties. All mints contain menthol, although some species contain more than others. Mints are especially healing for the mouth and teeth, making

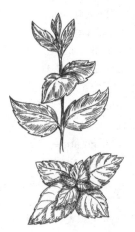

an excellent mouthwash. While Americans are usually most familiar with mint in sweet dishes, it is often used in more savory applications in Mediterranean cuisines. Try mint and cucumbers in yogurt dressing; it's delicious! Hot mint tea, which both heats and cools, is delightfully refreshing in both hot and cool weather and excellent for an upset stomach.

This refreshing quality extends to mint's magical uses. Mint is excellent in instances where things need to be cooled down, such as in antianxiety blends, or cast out, like sickroom blends. Mint is also excellent for other kinds of cleaning and clearing magic, particularly for curse breaking. The Haudenosaunee, for example, use it to cast out malicious witchcraft.[51] It can be used as an aspergillum for this purpose or be burned in cigars. It can also be burned over coals as an all-purpose cleanser, vibe improver, and to make a room smell good. Where I grew up, this sort of use would be said to be "just for nice." It is used in this way by almost every culture that has a relationship with a mint.

One Greek myth tells how the nymph Minthe was beloved of Hades, the god of death. When Persephone found out, she grew jealous and trampled Minthe underfoot. I believe, although I cannot prove, that this story began as an explanation of the custom of strewing mint along funeral paths—probably to cover the smell of the body. Mint was most certainly used in other ways in Greek funeral practices. This points to Mint's excellence as a necromancy ally. She makes open the way to and from the Land of the Dead. When combined with rose, mint is an excellent psychopomp; she helps make a path for those deceased who need assistance finding their way. Similarly, rose and mint together are excellent for healing grief; they clear a way back to life for the grieving. The same combination is excellent for healing a broken heart and for love magic more generally. Mint can also be used alone for improving a broken relationship; it is employed for this purpose among the Cheyenne.[52]

The most familiar mints to Americans are peppermint, spearmint, and apple mint, which, for the purposes of incense, are mostly interchangeable. When you can responsibly wildcraft it, native mint (*Mentha canadensis*) can also be used. It has a stronger smell than most European mints, so apply a little less. Also important medicinally and magically is the witch-plant and abortifacient pennyroyal, which I do not recommend for incense.

CATNIP

Catnip, *Nepeta cataria*, is a type of European mint. While it is not native anywhere in the United States, it is naturalized in most of the East. It is easy to grow, but be careful to keep it contained; it can take over. Cats, skunks, and butterflies all love it, but many insects do not. Like most insect-repellent plants, it can also be used to keep away spiritual pests.

Catnip's smoke is calming and mildly trance-inducing. Catnip is anxiolytic,* but its effects in this regard are somewhat stronger; it lets your cares float away. It can also produce, in some people, a sense of warm tingling in the body and mild euphoria. As always, these effects are very subtle in incense. Catnip can also be smoked from a pipe for a stronger effect. Catnip is excellent in spells to draw love, particularly for those wishing to draw men. It is also good to promote friendship and harmony among those who live together. Like most pollinator-attracting plants, catnip is good in offering incense for the Fair Folk and other helpful nature spirits. In most incense, catnip can often be replaced by damiana with a tiny amount of mint.

LEMON BALM

Lemon balm (*Melissa officinalis*) is a mint cousin native to the Mediterra-nean but naturalized throughout North America. It grows bright-green, ser-rated leaves that look similar to mint and smell of herbal lemon. The flow-ers are white, sometimes pale yellow or lavender. It is extremely easy to grow and should be contained if you do not want it to invade. Remove the

---

*   That is, it can be used to treat anxiety.

flowers before they go to seed. As the genus name *Melissa** indicates, this is a preferred plant for honeybees and many other pollinators, but it repels mosquitoes and many other pest insects. Like all pest-repelling herbs, it can be used as a light banisher. For this purpose, I find the best way to employ it is fresh, as an aspergillum. Lemon balm has long been used as a strewing herb. In the 19th century, it was often laid in the aisles between church pews. It can be burned as a single-note incense, but the scent is better from the fresh leaves. Lemon balm makes a delightful tea; I prefer it iced.

In incense, lemon balm is almost always uplifting; it brings a pleasant, mellow, solar energy. It is particularly nice for lifting grief and making the heart merry. It is often used in love magic to keep things from turning too angsty and dramatic. It can also be applied in sleep, dream, and trance work for its relaxing and soothing properties. For these uses, it's nice in the bath.

BASIL

Basil (*Ocimum basilicum*) is a familiar cooking herb and among the easiest herbs to grow yourself. It is so popularly cultivated, and for so long, that it is hard to pinpoint its origins, but basil almost certainly entered Europe from India; some say it was first imported by Alexander the Great. It can easily be rooted from fresh cuttings purchased at a grocery store and will flourish with little care in any sunny window or garden. Grocery store basil is generally the Italian (or sweet) variety. Asian basils are spicier and have pointier leaves. Basils are not winter-hardy in the north; you should either bring them in or plant a new one in the spring. Basil is an excellent companion plant for tomatoes; they are both strengthened when grown near each other. When in flower, basil is well favored by pollinators and also by the Good Neighbors. When used for magic, basil should never be cut with an iron blade; doing so will make the stem turn black. For incense purposes, all basils can be used interchangeably unless you wish to work with the spirit of one specific plant.

Tulsi, or holy basil (*Ocimum tenuiflorum*), is a closely related plant native to the Indian subcontinent. The plant is an avatar of the goddess Lakshmi, who showers her beloved in wealth and luxury and is a wife of Krishna. It is considered very lucky as a well-tended and revered houseplant. It can be brewed as a calming and warming tea, and some preliminary

---

*   Which is Latin for honeybee.

research suggests it may be helpful in treating inflammation and diabetes. Its taste is similar to basil mixed with black pepper.

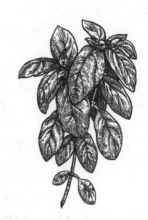

In addition to their deliciousness, basils are excellent magical allies. Like many highly aromatic plants, basil was used to dress the dead, and it can be burned as an incense to ease the passage of the recently deceased. In Wicca and derivative practices, basil is often used for wealth magic. One simple spell is to carry a fresh basil leaf in your wallet to attract money. Replace it each week, ideally on Thursday. Basil is also often used in spells to attract a new lover. Basil helps promote family harmony; for this purpose, it is most easily administered in food. It is excellent as a purifying incense, either alone or in concert with other ingredients, and also makes a good purifying bath. It can be used as a purifying scrub in the shower if you do not have a bathtub big enough to soak in. For this purpose, I combine it with salt, olive oil, and a little honey. It can also be used, with holy water, as an aspergillus to cleanse a room.

In ancient Greece, basil was associated with hatred and warfare, and it was thought best to sow its seeds while cursing the plant in anger, but I do not understand the origins of this custom. To determine who has cursed you, slowly throw basil leaves into a fire while naming your suspects. The basil indicates guilt when it makes a popping noise. It can also be burned as an incense to dispel malefica.

OREGANOS

Oreganos are a large family of highly fragrant flowering perennials native to the Mediterranean and surrounding areas. In lore, it is difficult to distinguish between regular oregano (*Origanum vulgare*), sweet marjoram (*O. majorana*), and Cretan dittany (*O. dictamnus*); the same names were used for all of them. For the most part, they can be substituted one for the other in incense, although I am especially fond of dittany of Crete, which I will talk about in more detail below. The name *oregano* comes from the Greek *oreao* (mountains) and *ganos* (joy), and it was well favored by Greek herbalists, healers, and cooks. Like all healing herbs that grow in the mountains, it is sacred to Artemis. Some sources say that Artemis was depicted wearing a crown of oregano, but I have never seen such an image.

Oreganos placed by the bed while sleeping promote dreams of future lovers. Hanging marjoram over the door prevents unwanted visits from wicked witches, restless ghosts, goblins, and other undesirable spirits. One 16th-century herbal recommends it for many things, including to treat those "given to overmuch sighing" or "against the swouning of the heart."[53] In the Victorian language of flowers, oreganos signal joy, and that is their primary association for me as well.

In Sephardic traditions, marjoram, as well as other oreganos, is used extensively for healing, and the smoke is employed to divine the true nature and cause of illness. For a healing tonic called "al sereno" (night dew), fill a glass partly with water, honey, and marjoram, and leave it outside overnight. In the morning, filter it, and then say the following Ladino prayer before drinking it: *"Kon el nombre del Patron del Mundo, esto ke me sea me melezina"* ("In the name of the Master of the World, let this be my cure").[54]

Dittany of Crete

Dittany of Crete (*Origanum dictamnus*) is a type of small perennial oregano which is native only to the high mountain slopes of Crete, but now cultivated around the world. In Greek, it is called *diktamo*. Dittany is a vulnerable plant that doesn't grow well where I live, but I love it so much I import it. Be cautious with sourcing, both for ethical reasons and because commercial diktamo is sometimes fake. If you buy the herb online, be sure you're getting whole leaves and that they are fuzzy and gray. Two different sellers have sent me oregano when I ordered dittany of Crete.

Diktamo has a long history of use on Crete, for medicinal and magical applications. Saved seeds were found in the ancient Minoan palace of Knossos, indicating its cultivation likely stretches back into prehistory. It is often brewed as a medicinal tea, usually to treat digestive issues. Although it is a common flavoring in liquors such as vermouth, it is rarely cooked with. It tastes strongly medicinal. In the local Cretan dialect, it is called *erontas,* which simply means "of Eros." Young men brave the cliffs to gather it for their sweethearts, and it is very efficacious in love spells.

Many people say that diktamo's name derives from the goddess Diktynna, a goddess in the court of Artemis and Hekate, who gave the gift of hunting and fishing nets to men. Diktynna was also a midwife in attendance to Rhea as she birthed Zeus. Certainly, my experience is that Hekate quite likes diktamo, and the smell clearly evokes the lonely mountains Artemis so adores. However, it is more likely that both the herb and the goddess are named after Mount Dikti, the Cretan mountain on whose slopes it grows, where the infant Zeus was hidden from his murderous father by the nanny goat Amalthea.

However, diktamo's most famed ancient magical use is in healing. For example, In the *Aeneid*, Venus heals Aeneas with dittany: "Hereupon Venus, smitten by her son's cruel pain, with a mother's care plucks from Cretan Ida a dittany stalk, clothed with downy leaves and purple flowers; not unknown is that herb to wild goats, when winged arrows have lodged in their flanks."[55]

In Greek folklore both ancient and modern, diktamo is famed for its potency as a necromantic herb. It is said to help promote peaceful and happy sleep among the dead; to find it growing on a grave indicates the spirit is joyful. In more modern times, diktamo was favored by both Helena Blavatsky and Aleister Crowley, who recommended it for producing trance, journey, and vision, as well as in evocation smoke. I use it in that way as well, and find it is particularly good for work involving travel in time.

THYME

Thyme (genus *Thymus*) is another genus of herbs in the Lamiaceae family, closely related to the oreganos. Its origins are clouded by history. It appears to be native to the Eastern Mediterranean but is now grown all over the world. Thyme is a common kitchen herb, so if you cook, you're certainly familiar with it. If not, you might know it as the warm, earthy, herbal taste of Thanksgiving stuffing, herbes de Provence, or Arabian za'atar.

Thyme is an abortifacient, although not an especially effective one. It is better for inducing labor in full-term pregnancies. For this reason, thyme is sacred to Birthgivers, Midwife Goddesses, and Witch Queens. Thyme was often strewn in medieval birthing beds to ease and speed labor. Perhaps to teach this practice, folk stories tell that the straw in the manger in which Jesus was born

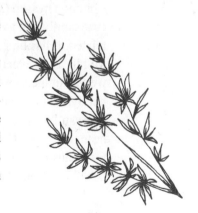

was strewn with wild thyme. It is sometimes called "Our Lady's Bedstraw" for this reason.

Thyme was used by Egyptians as an embalming herb and continued to be employed as a funeral incense and coffin stuffing well into the Middle Ages. In Wales, it is planted on graves.[56] It has a long history of being burned as a fumigant to rid a space of restless ghosts, and I recommend it with frankincense for this purpose. Thyme is excellent as an all-purpose incense and popular this way throughout Russia and Eastern Europe. In fact, the English word *thyme* derives from the same roots as the Greek word θυμίαμα (*thymiama*), which means "incense." Thyme was a favorite temple incense in ancient Greece. It was also popular in Greek magic to increase courage; the Greek word θύμος (*thymos*) means both "thyme" and "courage." In Rome, to say someone "smelled of thyme" meant you thought they were very brave. In the Middle Ages, knights about to joust wore sprigs of thyme or scarves embroidered with bee and thyme, given to them by ladies who favored them.[57]

Thyme is also very strongly associated with the Queens of the Wood and the Good Neighbors. Like most plants favored by them, it is also beloved by honeybees. In the British Isles, it is said that the dew that collects on thyme leaves the morning of the first of May has magical properties. If you wash your eyes with it, you will be able to see the Fair Folk. Shakespeare has Titania, the Queen of Fairies, make her bed in "a bank where the wild thyme blows . . ."[58] You should consider doing the same; the use of thyme as a strewing herb around the bed is said to prevent nightmares.

HYSSOP

Common hyssop (*Hyssopus officinalis*) is a tall shrubby herb in the Lamiaceae family that looks a little bit like tarragon, although they are not closely related. It has pink or blue flowers. It is native to southern Europe and the Middle East, where it has a long history of use in magic and healing, as well as in incense. However, the biblical hyssop was likely not this plant, but Syrian oregano (*Origanum syriacum*). For the purposes of incense, the two can be used interchangeably. In the magic of the Eastern Mediterranean, including Greece, Egypt, and the Levant, hyssop is extensively used for cleansing and protection, as in Psalm 51:7: "Purge me with hyssop, and I shall be clean; Wash me, and I shall be whiter than snow." In these cases,

Syrian oregano is best, but if it cannot be had, a mixture of common hyssop, thyme, and dittany of Crete (or another oregano) is a good substitute.

SAGE & OTHER SALVIAS

Salvia is a large genus of plant, all part of the broader mint (Lamiaceae) family. As you can tell from the name, these plants are excellent healing allies. Nearly all members of the *Salvia* genus are healers—some of the body and some of the more ephemeral maladies of mind, spirit, and soul. Salvias, as a rule, are extremely good pollinators, drawing bees and butterflies to the garden, along with other Good Neighbors. One of the defining characteristics of salvias is their unusual pollination mechanism. Salvias do not easily cross-pollinate, which leads to a very wide variety of forms, each adapted to its own particular habitat. Salvia, as a spirit teacher, can teach us to do the same. It helps support the mental and spiritual flexibility to blossom into something new when you need to, without giving up on the core features that make you *you*. This same adaptability means that the genus is a very wide category, including plants that at first appear very different.

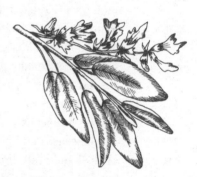

Common Sage

Salvia officinalis, called common, garden, or kitchen sage, is native to the Mediterranean, but has been cultivated worldwide for millennia. Common sage is an evergreen perennial shrub in its native climate. There are many varieties, most of which have broad, soft, grayish-green leaves with soft hairs. Some more ornamental cultivars tend toward yellow or purple. It is readily identified by its familiar spicy herbal smell. It is extremely easy to grow in many climates, favoring hot, dry locations. While it can be raised from seed or cuttings, it's also easy to buy small seedlings. It needs to be cut back each autumn; otherwise the plant will become woody and not grow as well.

Sage is a healing herb par excellence, as the Latin proverb would have it: *"Cur moriatur homo, ciu salvia crescit in horto"* or "Why would a person die, if they have sage in their garden?" Common sage was a foundational plant in medieval European gardens and apothecaries; it was used in a variety of culinary applications, as well as medical ones. Even stronger is the Old English proverb "He that would live for aye* must eat sage in May."

Brewed as a tea, it is used as a diuretic and tonic, and as a healing skin wash. It is also said to be good for the teeth and gums. Many people rinse their hair with sage tea to make it shiny and healthy and to prevent graying. According to one 16th-century British herbal, it "is singularly good for the head and brain, it quickeneth the senses and memory, strengtheneth the sinews, restoreth health to those that have the palsy, and taketh away shakey trembling of the members."[59] I recommend sage tea with lemon and honey for sore throats. Consult a doctor or herbalist before using sage tea if you are breastfeeding and wish to continue doing so; it can slow milk production.

Although the use of the word *sage* to mean "wise elder" is not etymologically related to the plant's name, sage is an excellent tonic for the mind. It is said to improve memory and focus and to prevent cognitive decline in the elderly. There is some very limited clinical research to support sage's benefit to Alzheimer's patients, although further studies are needed.[60] Sage's close cousin rosemary, as we'll discuss below, is even better for memory.

As an incense, sage is most often used to warm and comfort and to lift the senses and improve mental acuity. It is good for depression, both clinical and mild. It can also be used to purify or banish. It is particularly good at clearing miasma from the sickroom, although I do not recommend any kind of incense be burned around people with respiratory illnesses. Instead, in those cases, burn the incense in the room while the sick person is elsewhere and allow the smell to settle, or use the herbs in steam. Sage is also a good herb to add to all types of warming or soothing incenses; its connection with holiday foods gives it an air of home and family.

Clary Sage

Salvia sclarea, called clary (or clear-eye) sage, is a Mediterranean salvia that is today primarily cultivated for its fragrance, although historically it was also an important medicinal herb. It is also used to flavor certain liqueurs. It is easy to grow in many climates but can be invasive; use caution and do some research about your local ecosystem before planting it.

---

*   That is, forever.

Clary sage is similar in smell to most sages, although slightly more medicinal and with a pronounced stanky/musky undertone. In small doses, it is pleasant enough, but it can be overpowering when too much is employed. Today, it is most frequently used in essential oil form as a fragrance fixative and in the production of artificial ambergris, a historical scent produced in the intestines of sperm whales.

White Sage

When people talk about burning sage, they almost always mean white sage, or *Salvia apiana* (bee sage). It is so named because it is an important attractor of pollinators, especially carpenter bees. Like most pollinator plants, it is beloved by the Good Neighbors.

White sage is native to the southwestern United States and northwestern Mexico. I am told it is easy to grow in warm climates (zones 8–11), but it will not overwinter where I live. In its native region, it is used medicinally, religiously, and magically by many indigenous peoples. For example, the Cahuilla (Ivilyuqaletem) people of southern California eat and smoke the leaves (both in pipes and in sweat lodge ceremonies) and use it as a deodorant. Additionally, they rub it on their bodies before hunting to disguise natural human odors, including those of menstruating women.[61] Among the Kumeyaay (Diegueño), it is burned as an incense or suffumigation, particularly in the sickroom, especially when there has been measles in the home.[62] In many cases, people in the native range of both use blue sage (*Artemisia tridentata*) interchangeably for white.

Sloppily appropriated from indigenous practices, "smudging," or suffumigation with white sage, has become popular in modern Anglophone paganism. It is often done in one of two ways. In the first style, loose dried leaves are burned over charcoal in an abalone shell and wafted with a feather fan. In the other, white sage is partly dried and then wrapped into cigars. Many people, including me, consider these practices culturally appropriative. Out of respect for indigenous people and their sacred traditions, the word *smudging* should not be applied to nonindigenous incense practices.

Because of this nonindigenous use, and the commodification thereof, white sage has become chronically overharvested, although it is not endangered. Take care when sourcing this material and grow your own if possible. If you are not growing your own and building a relationship with the living spirit of the plant, I recommend against its use outside of traditional indigenous ceremony. For most applications, mugwort and rosemary can be substituted for white sage.

ROSEMARY

Rosemary (*Salvia rosmarinus*) was only recently (2017) reclassified into the *Salvia* genus; it is different from other salvias in some important ways. Doubtless, the spicy, slightly medicinal smell and taste of rosemary are familiar to you; it's a common kitchen herb. As with all salvias, it is an excellent pollinator and a friend to the Good Neighbors. As one 19th-century herbal says, "The young fairies, under the guise of snakes, lie concealed under its branches."[63] Rosemary is evergreen in its native Mediterranean habitat and has small needlelike leaves. In sunny locations out of the wind, it will overwinter here in zone 6, but I doubt it could survive much farther north. The plant's name in ancient days was *ros marinus*, the dew of the sea, because it thrives by the sea. However, a popular folk etymology makes it the Rose of Mary, and relates the following story:

> On the road to Bethlehem, the very pregnant Mary was caught in a rainstorm, and sought shelter under an evergreen bush, spreading her light blue cloak out over the strong branches, and making herself a bed of the needles. In the morning, the aura of her holiness had permeated the whole plant, leaving them with her own spicy-sweet smell, and the blue dye had soaked from her cloak into the flowers, and that is why Mary's rose has flowers of such a beautiful and delicate blue.

Rosemary is most famously associated with memory. As Shakespeare would have Ophelia say: "There's rosemary, that's for remembrance; pray, love, remember."[64] Rosemary has millennia of documented use for memory. Students in ancient Greece found it effective to wear wreaths of it while taking exams. This efficacy is also supported by several modern studies. In his *Herball*, Roger Hacket said: "It helpeth the brain, strengtheneth the memorie, and is very medicinable for the head."[65] It has also been shown to be effective in some older adults to improve memory and general cognitive function, a practice documented in folklore since antiquity.

Because of its association with the seashore, and the beauty of its appearance and smell, rosemary is often linked to the goddess Aphrodite. Perhaps because of this association, rosemary is an excellent choice for magical work dealing with marriage, whether you are looking to marry or working to improve the marriage you are already in. Brides in many European cultures have traditionally worn crowns of rosemary. Rosemary is particularly famed for its use in fidelity work. Feed your spouse rosemary and place a sprig of it in their pocket to keep them faithful. To "spice things up" in the bedroom, use seven knots of red thread to tie together three sprigs of rosemary and a cinnamon stick, and put the bundle under your bed. This is also said to help keep away bedbugs and other insects.

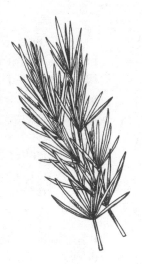

Because of its anti-insect and antimicrobial properties, you should suspect that rosemary will have protective and banishing qualities, and folklore bears this out. Rosemary wreaths on a door keep away unwanted visitors, particularly those on "official" business. Rosemary is an excellent fumigation for the sickroom, and rosemary-scented steam is good for those with colds and other respiratory illnesses. Because of its antimicrobial action, rosemary is customary in funeral rites nearly everywhere it has naturalized. Rosemary is also a strongly protective herb, useful for warding off curses and other malefica. The needles are often used in witch-bottles and other apotropaic folk magic to represent pins, blades, and pointy things. It can also be used to ward off nightmares. Rosemary is excellent in the bath; whole sprigs can be added, or you can brew a strong tea to pour over yourself in the shower. Bathing in rosemary is a good restorative and can help improve the circulation.

Rosemary is also a very strong ally in the fight against the patriarchy. An Old English saying goes: "Where rosemary grows, the woman is master." Magically, it is an excellent choice in poppets of abusers, where its needles poke and prod, making it impossible for them to forget what they have done. As a wash, it helps bruises heal. In tea, it helps to calm the heart and mind, particularly after trauma.

In incense, rosemary can be used for all of the above purposes. When burned alone, it is almost always a banisher and purifier, particularly of illness and malefica. In combination with other elements, rosemary is excellent as a clarifier, sweeping away any magical clutter that might work against the other ingredients. It is good in offerings for Aphrodite, Juno, and the Good Neighbors, although it makes a better offering in combination with softer and rounder scents, like frankincense. On its own, rosemary is very clear, sharp, and bright, like a shiny sword.

SEER'S SAGE

It would be disingenuous to write a chapter about salvia incenses without discussing *Salvia divinorum*, also called "diviner's sage" or "ska María pastora" (plant of Mary the shepherdess*), or most frequently, simply "salvia." This salvia is a psychotropic plant native to Oaxaca. It has known millennia of continuous use by the indigenous people of that region, including the modern Mazatec, as a teacher plant, to facilitate trance and spirit journeying, primarily in the context of divinatory and healing ritual.[66] Its use was popularized among nonindigenous people largely through the work of Albert Hofmann, who studied it late in his career. *Salvia divinorum*, like many domesticated plants, very rarely reproduces from seed, thus very few genetically distinct plants are known. Almost all salvia you will ever encounter is cloned from one of two cuttings from Oaxaca. One was made in 1962 and is called the Wasson-Hofmann strain. It is also sometimes called the bitter strain because of its bad taste. The other was cut in 1991 and is called the Blosser or palatable strain.

For entheogenic work, salvia is generally consumed as tea, but it can also be smoked or used as incense. Obviously, you should exercise extreme caution when working with salvia or any other entheogen. I recommend only learning this work in person, from an experienced trance worker who shows appropriate respect to the traditions and spirits involved. Salvia is dangerous when not worked with properly. It is illegal in many countries including the UK and Australia; however, it is legal in most (but not all) U.S. states.

---

* *Pastora*, which I have translated "shepherd," can also mean "guide," "priest," or "shaman."

Other Herbs

VERVAIN

Vervain (also called verbena) is a large family of plants. For the purposes of incense, they are generally interchangeable, with a few exceptions that I'll discuss below. All vervains are sacred to the Queen of Heaven; I find this especially true of the blue-flowered varieties. In Egypt, this plant was called "tears of Isis," and in Greece it was sacred to Hera and Eos, the dawn. All vervains attract pollinators, particularly bees and butterflies, and are excellent for work with the Fair Folk. Verbenas are common in love magic, as well as for protection and healing. Medicinally, vervain is a relaxant, and magically its use follows suit. It is excellent in any work designed to calm and diffuse the flow of energy, both internal and external. Among its most famous uses in magic is as the basis for vanvan oil, which is usually made from lemon verbena. In fact, the word *vanvan* is a Creole variant on the word *verbena*.

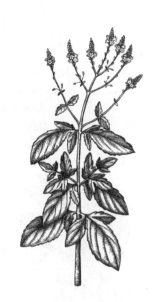

The most common types for incense making are common vervain (*Verbena officinalis*), which is native to Europe, and blue vervain, also called American vervain (*Verbena hastata*). Also of note is another American native, hoary verbena (*Verbena stricta*), and the South American lemon verbena (*Aloysia citrodora*). These varieties can all be interchanged in incense, but, of course, they each have their own special qualities.

DAMIANA

Damiana, *Turnera diffusa*, has a complex spicy, floral scent, somewhat reminiscent of chamomile. Closely related to passionflower, it also has a great reputation as an aphrodisiac. Its name comes from the Greek *daman*, which means "to subdue" (as with a love spell). When burned, damiana has a dank herbal scent, similar to marijuana mixed with fruit. Damiana can be smoked from a pipe and is frequently blended with marijuana. Smoked damiana produces a smooth, mild, and pleasant body high as well as very mild euphoria. It can also function as an anxiolytic. The effect in incense is the same, but much subtler. In Mexico, it is brewed into a traditional liquor, which was the original base of margaritas. The brand with which I am familiar comes in a splendid fat goddess-shaped bottle.

Magically, damiana is excellent in all sorts of work relating to love or sex. It is a strong aphrodisiac in people of all sexes, but particularly in those with vaginas. It is also a good aid in divination, trance, and dream work. So associated is it with trance journeying that it has the witchiest traditional name in this book: "Old Woman's Broom." In most incenses, it can be substituted with a combination of catnip and mugwort.

BAY LAUREL

Bay laurel (*Laurus nobilis*) is a Mediterranean shrub, evergreen with slick black drupes. The leaves are smooth, shiny, and shaped like spearpoints. They smell sharply herbal, with floral and citrus elements. They are a common flavoring agent in soups, stews, and sauces. Bay laurel is a common

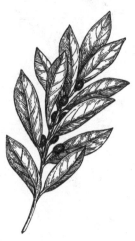

garden plant in warm climates and often grown indoors. Some say that keeping a bay laurel in the house will prevent lightning from striking your home. The native California bay (*Umbellularia californica*) is not the same plant, but it can be used interchangeably in incense. California bay tends to be stronger, so use less.

Bay leaves are excellent protection against pantry moths and many other pests. This hints to us that they are also protective against discorporate pests, and my experience bears this out. Bay is an excellent banisher, particularly against the restless dead. With frankincense, it makes an excellent curse-breaker. When an unwanted guest finally leaves, fumigate with bay smoke to keep them from coming back. Finally, in a trick I learned from Caroline Kenner of Gryphons Grove School of Shamanism, bay is a powerful martial ally in the Other Place. Shape-shift into a bay laurel tree, and spin around as a multiarmed warrior, using each of your leaves as a knife.

The Greek name for the bay laurel is *Δάφνη*, or *daphne*, named for a nymph Apollo chased. In days long past, Eros laid a curse upon Apollo. Driven mad by lust, he chased the naiad Daphne, intent on rape. Just before he caught her, she cried out to Gaia for help, who intervened and turned Daphne into a tree. Ovid recounts the scene thus: "Heavy numbness seized her limbs, thin bark closed over her breast, her hair turned into leaves, her arms into branches, her feet so swift a moment ago stuck fast in slow-growing roots, her face was lost in the canopy. Only her shining beauty was left."[67] Apollo wove himself a wreath of her beautiful branches, and her powerful magic exorcised the curse that was on him. For this reason, bay is said to be very sacred to Apollo. As with most myths of this type, this came into being to explain an existing practice, not the other way round. Bay is sacred to Apollo because it is sacred to Delphi, whose slopes it covers. Bay is sacred to Apollo because it so loves the sun. Bay is sacred to Apollo because it is bright and crisp and clear. The sacredness of bay vastly predates the invention of Apollo.

Bay leaves were said to be huffed by the oracles at Delphi,[68] and they are excellent in all divination incense. Bay leaves can also be used as a potpourri; place them next to your bed to promote true dreaming. A common practice in modern Anglophone folk magic is to write things from which you wish to be released on bay leaves and then burn them. Others write wishes on the leaves, and burn them as an offering to the sun. If you have access to whole plants, the drupes and wood can also be added to incense. Bay laurel incense is both bacteriocidal and fungicidal; it is an excellent fumigation for the sickroom.

CONIFER NEEDLES

The needles of almost all conifers can be burned as incense and are largely interchangeable, except in cases where you are working directly with the spirit of the tree. More or less all conifer needles smell pleasant when burned, and all are good for purification. I most commonly use pine, juniper, and cypress, all of which we've already discussed. Fir is particularly good for building inner confidence and spiritual authority. It is used both ceremonially and more mundanely as an incense among many indigenous peoples of North America. Spruce is said to improve the psychic senses and open the mind to clarity. Yew needles are poisonous in large quantities but are still sometimes burned for malefica. Use appropriate caution when experimenting.

WAIT! WHAT ABOUT LAVENDER?

Those of you familiar with magical herbs might be surprised that none of the recipes in this book involve lavender. There's a simple explanation: I'm allergic to it! I'm not comfortable recommending magic I've never worked myself, and that's why it's not included. Because I don't grow, ingest, or work with lavender, I can't tell you much more about it than you would learn from Wikipedia. It's an herb of the same Lamiaceae family we discussed above. It has lovely, very fragrant light-purple flowers that attract pollinators. It is especially famed for its calming and sleep-bringing properties. I can't use it, but almost every other witch I know loves it. I encourage you to experiment with lavender.

Flowers

Rose

Roses are among the most well-known and culturally significant ingredients in this book, and so I won't waste too much time in describing them. I'm confident you know what roses look and smell like. If you'd like information about growing them, there are many sources far better than I am! Instead, let's look a bit into their history, and then we'll delve right into discussing their use in magical incenses.

There are many species of wild roses, most of which have five petals. When pollinated, most produce a type of fruit called a rose hip. These hips are sour but delicious and very high in vitamin C. I recommend brewing a tea of them. In domesticated varieties like you find at a florist or a fancy garden, the petals are so numerous and tight that the flowers usually can't pollinate without human assistance, and so they do not form hips. For this reason, if using rose in a mixture for fertility, I recommend either wild roses or rose hips along with domesticated ones. Be cautious not to use florist rose petals in incense you expect to huff; they're often covered in pesticides.

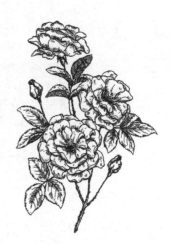

One myth tells of the rose's origins: Flora, the Goddess of Spring and of Flowers, one day found the dead body of her best beloved nymph. Inconsolable, she begged all the gods to come to her aid to change the body of her dear one into the most beautiful flower, which would be recognized as Queen of all Flowers. "Apollo, God of the Arts, gave her the breath of life. Bacchus bathed her in nectar. Vertumnus gave her fragrance, Pomona her fruit, and Flora herself finally gave a diadem of petals, and thus the rose was born."[69]

Roses are renowned for their beauty and delicious smell; they are the quintessential sensual delight. They demand the attention of all who see them. For this reason, they are excellent for all magic that involves catching the eye of someone else, whether for romance, employment, or any other reason. However, roses are, of course, especially good for love, sex, and romance-drawing magic. I recommend red rose petals for sex, pink for love, white for marriage, yellow for friendship, and orange for employment. While any color of rose petals is excellent for any of these uses, you can specialize a mixture further by concentrating on color. Personally, I usually have only red roses "in stock," but I save all the rose petals that come my way. Roses given lover to lover are especially effective in magic targeting that relationship.

Roses are the emblem of Venus, the goddess of love, and a key ingredient in almost any offering incense for her or other spirits in her sphere. Many, many other deities adore roses, including Inanna, Ishtar, Aphrodite, Lakshmi, Chloris, Cybele, Flora, Demeter, Astarte, Aurora, Hekate, Cupid, Dionysus, Eros, Mars, and Bacchus. All works attended by those spirits are aided by rose incense.

Roses are excellent in healing magic, particularly emotional healing. They add a calming, restorative action to any blend. Additionally, roses are an excellent offering for the dead. In ancient Greek folklore, the body of Hector, the great warrior prince, was anointed in rose oil after he fell, to show his might in the afterlife. Finally, roses are excellent at dispelling the evil eye; it is wise to include them in protective magic, especially for children. This is the mirror of roses' attractive function; by attracting attention and making you look awesome, roses can also make you prone to the evil eye. However, as always, the poison is also the cure, when used in the right way, and rose is an excellent ally in curse-breaking work. Finally, rose hips, fresh from the plant, are covered in tiny itchy hairs; in fact, you can grind them up to make itching powder. For this reason, they are also an excellent addition to certain kinds of bane work.

Jasmine

The name *jasmine* is commonly applied to many kinds of flowering plants, but when purchased commercially or used in incense, it generally refers to *Jasminum odoratissimum*, also called "sweet-smelling jasmine," or *Cestrum nocturnum*, called "night-blooming jasmine" or "Queen of the Night." Jasmine flowers are small, white, star-shaped, and very strongly scented. The flowers are sometimes brewed with tea, especially in China. Like rose, it has a very strongly floral smell common in feminine perfumes.

Jasmine has an aura of sadness about it as well. In Filipino legend, it is associated with a pair of star-crossed lovers. A prince and a peasant girl fell in love. She worried to him, "You will forget me in the morning. I am only a plain country girl, with no fancy jewels or perfumes. I have only this jasmine in my hair." He told her he could never be unfaithful to her and handed her his dagger, "Should I ever betray you, stab me in the heart with this blade." The prince rode off once more to his palace, and (of course) forgot all about the country girl and her jasmine flower.

Time passed, and the country girl heard of the prince's impending marriage to a fine, rich, city woman. She traveled many days to the city and slipped into the wedding crowd unnoticed. But she could not bring herself to stab the prince. Instead, she went to her beloved jasmine bush and carved his name into the bush, with the words "I bow to you." Then, she stabbed herself. Her blood fed and awakened the bush, which grew huge and more perfumed than any other. To this day, it is said, if two lovers inhale jasmine together, they will be caught up in a love drama no one can resist.

Magically, jasmine is closely associated with the night sky, and also with femininity and motherhood in many cultures. It is thought of as a purifying force and often used as a lunar herb. In incense, jasmine primarily lends luxury and romance and enhances and clarifies psychic vision. However, as you can tell from the story above, it is not always a wise addition. A bowl of jasmine flowers near the bed, or their inclusion in an herbal pillow, is said to promote prophetic dreaming, although I prefer star anise for this purpose.

Clover

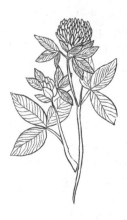

Clover is an amazing and beautiful magical plant. As a genus, *Trifolium* is what's called "cosmopolitan"; that is, it is native or naturalized in nearly every ecoregion of the Earth. Its three-leafed "shamrock" shape, which St. Patrick associated with the trinity, to me speaks to clover's cosmopolitanism; she is native not just to all the Earth, but to the Heavens and Underworld as well. My personal experience is with Dutch white clover (*Trifolium repens*) and red clover (*Trifolium pratense*), both of which grow in my yard, and probably yours too. Of the two, my experience is that white clover is slightly better for working with the Fair Folk, and red clover is better for healing, but for incense all clovers are pretty much the same. Clover can be grown indoors, but I have always been taught that to do so is unlucky.

In Christian lore, each of the leaves represents a magical virtue: the first is trust, the second hope, the third love, and the fourth leaf, when it appears, represents luck. It's widely believed that four-leaf clovers, on average, appear on about 1/10,000 clovers. If they were distributed randomly, that's about one four-leaf clover per a twelve-square-foot area. However, the four-leaf mutation is inheritable, and so once there is one four-leaf clover, there are likely to be more nearby. Personally, I am quite confident that magical/fairy activity tends to mutate clovers toward the four-leaf varieties. Here's a tip to help you find them: White clover has white splotches on the leaves that on normal clovers form a triangle. On four-leafers, they create a square. Look for the squares among triangles. If you find a four-leafer, you might want to collect the flowers from it after they bloom and just begin to turn brown and specially nurture those seeds. In Cornwall, they say that an ointment can be made from four-leaf clovers to promote the second sight, although I have not had success with this. In Wales, four-leaf clovers are placed under the pillow to promote magical dreaming, good health, and a cheerful mood.[70] Four-leaf clovers picked on May Day are especially lucky.

Clover is an important pollination plant, particularly for bees, who adore it. It is a favored food for rabbits, groundhogs, and other small mammals, as well as deer. Like almost all plants favored by pollinators, it is also favored by the Fair Folk. Planting it will attract beneficent spirits and keep away malefic ones. I strongly associate clover with the Great Goddess, Heavy with Child, partly because it contains high quantities of phytoestrogens. Clovers sequester far more carbon and produce far more oxygen per acre than regular grass does. They also fix nitrogen in the soil to nourish the land. One very easy thing you can do to re-wild the world is to over-seed clover into your lawn and allow it to flower; this not only promotes enchantment and spirit diversity, it restores the fertility of despoiled land, encourages pollinator populations, and reduces water waste.

Clover is also excellent for wealth-drawing magic. In fact the phrase "living in the clover" is an old-fashioned way to say "living a life of luxury." I believe this to be because, as I mentioned above, clover makes the soil very healthy and is also excellent fodder for grazing animals, so farms rich in clover are rich farms indeed. Clover blossoms sprinkled on the doorstep of a business are said to attract customers. It can also be used in a bath to wash away bad money luck and draw prosperity. In modern Greek folk practice, clover is used to asperge the corners of a room, especially a sickroom, with vinegar. This drives away demons. For incense, I use primarily the flowers, although I occasionally also include the leaves. Clover flower has a light floral fragrance that, to me, is the smell of summer.

Saffron

Saffron, the bright yellow stigmas (reproductive parts) of the *Crocus sativus* flower, was domesticated from wild autumn crocus (*Crocus cartwrightianus*), which is native in the Attic Peninsula, Crete, and Asia Minor. It's unclear where it was first domesticated but it has been propagated by humans across Eurasia since at least the Bronze Age and is now grown worldwide. Today almost 90 percent of the world's saffron is produced in Iran. In the Americas, little saffron is farmed except by the Pennsylvania Deitsch, particularly those of Lancaster, Pennsylvania.*

Because harvesting the stigmas is extremely labor-intensive, saffron is very expensive and has always been so. It takes seventy thousand crocuses to produce a pound of saffron. Saffron produces a bright yellow color when

---

* Where I grew up.

cooked, especially in rice. It is also used as a dye, although most cloth described as "saffron dyed" is actually colored with turmeric. Saffron has a smell that is difficult to describe. It is something like honey mixed with freshly mown hay—buttery and rich, without being creamy or sweet. It's very mildly spicy, but not at all hot. It's almost impossible to describe, but very delicious. There is a long history of saffron being used in perfumes and incense. Alexander the Great and Cleopatra are both said to have bathed in it; it is famed for promoting both beauty and wound healing.

There is some evidence that saffron can reduce symptoms in those with major depressive disorders. In my opinion it's hard to believe anything so yellow and so delicious wouldn't raise anyone's mood, at least a little! Magically, saffron is an excellent joy-bringer. Along this same vein, it is widely used to promote conviviality. It is a key ingredient in hippocras, a type of medieval mulled wine traditionally served as the final drink at banquets as a sort of farewell toast.

Saffron, in particular, and crocuses in general are sacred to Hermes. In Greek myth, Krokus was a lover of Hermes. Hermes accidentally killed him, and then created the saffron crocus to honor him. For this reason, saffron is often used in love-drawing magic by men seeking men. It is also sacred to Hekate and her god-daughter Kirke (Circe), the Witch Queen of Aeaea. In Egypt, saffron was beloved of Amun. Saffron is also sacred to many solar gods, almost certainly owing to its brilliant yellow color. It has a warm fiery energy; when used in incense, it is usually to bring a sense of luxury, comfort, and healing warmth.

Other Flowers

When used in small quantities, almost any flower can be added to incense. Experiment by burning a tiny bit of the dried flower by itself to see how it smells. Most flower petals have surprisingly little scent when burned, but they do add a lovely colorful element to loose incenses. Some add a delicate floral aroma. Many common garden flowers work well in incense; I often use daisies, dandelions, marigolds, hibiscus, violets, lilac, chrysanthemums, pansies, and sunflowers. Additionally, the flowers of any herbs you are using can be added with the leaves.

Spices, Seeds, Berries &
Other Fruits

WHILE THE WORD *herb* generally refers to the leaves or flowers of a plant, *spice* more often means the barks, seeds, and other "hard" constituents. However, there is some overlap between the categories. Their strong flavors and scents are the result of high concentrations of aromatic compounds, many of which have medicinal and magical value. Because spices are value-dense and shelf-stable, they were among the earliest Eastern goods imported into Europe, along the legendary Spice Road. Generally, most spices are good for martial and sexual magic or anything else where you want to add heat and "spice things up."

Pepper

Black pepper (*Piper nigrum*) is the most common spice in the world; I will not waste time describing its taste and smell, which you are surely familiar with. The part used is the small drupe, called a peppercorn. For magic, all colors of peppercorns can be interchanged; I usually use plain black peppercorns from the regular grocery store. Peppercorns were sometimes stuffed into the noses of corpses before mummification in ancient Egypt; like all mummification plants, I imagine they can be used in work with the dead, although I do not employ them that way.

In incense, pepper is generally used martially, usually in aggressive or malefic work. However, used sparingly, it can also bring a fiery martial edge to other kinds of magic as well. Because of its aggressiveness, pepper is most often used to drive things or people away; think of it like magical pepper spray. It can be added to general protective incenses, but be careful not to overdo it. For this purpose, it combines well with resins. Pepper is also good for alertness and wariness, especially before entering into literal or figurative battle. Add several peppercorns to spiced tea or coffee for a pick-me-up jolt when you need it. When traveling, or in another situation where ingredients are difficult to come by, mix the contents of a few packs of black pepper and salt. Sprinkle the mixture across the doorway for a quick and simple protective ward.

When used sparingly, pepper is an excellent fiery, martial, masculine addition to incenses related to love and sex; it spices things up and adds a hint of danger. It is excellent with roses and honey for that purpose. That same mixture also makes a good seasoning to feed to your beloved to put them "in the mood." *Warning:* Incense should use only whole peppercorns. *Do not* use ground or cracked pepper in incense; it smokes too fast and can irritate eyes, noses, and throats.

Vanilla

Vanilla (*Vanilla planifolia*) is a vine native to Mexico, but today commonly produced in Madagascar and Indonesia. Its bean-like seedpods are what we call vanilla. Like saffron, vanilla is expensive because it requires hand-pollination of the flowers, which die the day after they bloom. Because not

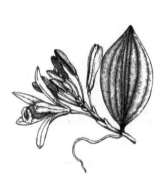

all the flowers bloom at the same time, nor do the fruits, both pollination and harvesting are very labor-intensive processes. Once the beans are harvested, they require months of curing. This is probably not a plant you can grow or wildcraft; however, it is easily available in most large grocery stores. Most commercial foods are made with artificial vanilla, which most people cannot distinguish from genuine vanilla when both are cooked. However, for magic, I strongly recommend using whole vanilla beans. When using vanilla in incense, split the beans open with a knife, and mix the tiny seeds into the other powdered ingredients. Put "empty" vanilla beans into a jar of sugar, where it will offer a subtle hint of its wonderful smell and flavor for everything you use the sugar in. Vanilla sugar is excellent for both baking and love spells. You can also use vanilla extract in incense. It's best to mix the liquid into honey first, and then mix the honey into the rest of the incense; otherwise, it is difficult to mix homogeneously.

Vanilla is an extremely common spice; I'm sure you know its smell well. It is warm, sweet, creamy, and very slightly piquant. It is a featured flavor in cookies, ice cream, and all sorts of other treats. For many of us, it smells like the very best childhood memories. Vanilla evokes feelings of simplicity and purity and is almost universally adored. While I'm sure there are people who don't like the smell of vanilla, I don't think I've ever met one. There is significant clinical evidence to support the claim that smelling vanilla reduces anxiety. This effect is true across all human cultures and also in animals, which indicates it is inherent to the plant itself, rather than being merely a reminder of happy times.

As far as we know, the Totonaca of central Mexico, who were later conquered and absorbed by the Aztec, were the first people to cultivate vanilla. They do not appear to have used it in food, but they did burn it ceremonially and employed it as an aphrodisiac. For example, young women wove the pods into their hair to attract lovers.[71] Modern Mexican Brujeria still uses it in much the same ways. A small piece of vanilla can be placed under the tongue when speaking to a love interest, or you can use a needle to thread the hair of your beloved through a bean.

German physician Bezaar Zimmermann, in his article "On Experiences" (1762), claimed: "No fewer than 342 impotent men, by drinking vanilla decoctions, had changed into astonishing lovers of at least as many women."[72] *King's American Dispensatory* teaches that vanilla "exhilarates the brain, prevents sleep, increases muscular energy, and stimulates the sexual propensities."[73] Indeed, vanilla is excellent in all types of love, sex, and romance magic and makes a lovely addition to almost any offering for love goddesses, as well as other spirits of the sphere of Venus. I have been known to spritz my sheets with it on nights when I expect company.

Cloves

Cloves (*Syzygium aromaticum*) are one of my very favorite spices. They are a favorite in Greek cooking, and to me, they smell like home. Cloves are excellent in magic. They can be used, like all luxury trade goods, in working to attract wealth and as offerings to the spirits of the sphere of

Jupiter. Like all spicy things, they can be added to love magic to "spice things up." Cloves are a traditional aphrodisiac that "gets the blood pumping." They can also be used as offerings to spirits of the sphere of Venus, although they are not my first choice for that. More specifically, cloves are good for attracting and nourishing friendships. To seal the deal, you and your friend should each tie seven cloves onto a red string. Exchange strings and wear them until they fall off. Cloves are also used in martial magic; often this magic directly draws on their shape, comparing them to spikes or weapons.

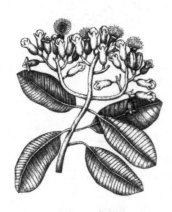

In Greek folk magic, cloves are used for both diagnosing and treating the evil eye. To diagnose, seven cloves are burned over a candle flame, one at a time. If they burn silently, all is well. The more popping there is, the worse the curse. In addition to their diagnostic use, cloves figure in a form of minor exorcism called ξεμάτιασμα (Xematiasma), which means something like "shake loose" or "shrug off." Xematiasma can be performed to cure the evil eye and can be executed in many ways. What I recommend is to brew a strong tea of cloves and add some salt. If this can be made with seawater, all the better. At the end of a shower, pour the salt-and-clove water over your head, while praying that you be cleansed and healed. Traditionally prayers for Xematiasma are a closely guarded secret; I cannot teach you my family's prayer. However, here are two I've written for you as examples to help you write your own:

Holy Virgin, Queen of Heaven,
Mother of God, Mother of All,
take us under your sky-blue cloak,
and protect us from all evil.
Avert, avert, avert!

Thea Euryphaessa, Queen of Heaven,
Holy Wide Shining One,
Mother of the Dawn, and the Moon,
and the ever-unconquered Sun,

Yours is the eternal Aithre; yours the clear blue sky,
Yours is the vision of prophecy, yours the all-seeing eye.
Shine your light upon this home,
And send all evil away to roam!
Avert, avert, avert!

In incense, cloves can also be used for protection from illness, insects, and unsavory magic. For this, they are excellent combined with mugwort and violets. However, I use them most often as luck-bringers and to excite spirits of a Mercurial bent. Cloves speed magical work up and bring a fiery power to energize almost any kind of magic. Clove smoke is "high vibration"; it rises above other smells and is a good choice in incenses that otherwise feel stale or heavy. Cloves, especially in concert with frankincense, are an excellent fumigation for sacred space.

Cinnamon & Cassia

True cinnamon (*Cinnamomum verum*), also called "Ceylon cinnamon," is a highly aromatic bark famed worldwide as a cooking spice. It is expensive, but easy to find in upscale grocery stores or specialty spice shops. In the United States, most grocery store cinnamon is Chinese cinnamon (*Cinnamomum cassia*), a closely related plant with similar bark, although other varieties are also used. For most purposes the two are interchangeable, although true cinnamon is definitely more delightful and delicious; I encourage you to try it if you have the opportunity to do so. In everything that follows, cinnamon refers to either variety.

Cinnamon has a long history of trade as a luxury good. In ancient days, its origins were shrouded in mystery in the west. Herodotus, in his *Histories*, writes: "Still more wonderful is the mode in which they collect the cinnamon. Where the wood grows, and what country produces it, they cannot tell—only some, following probability, relate that it comes from the country in which Bacchus was brought up. Great birds, they say, bring the sticks which we Greeks, taking the word from the Phoenicians, call cinnamon, and carry them up into the air to make their nests. These are fastened with a sort of mud to a sheer face of rock, where no foot of man is able to climb. So the Arabians, to get the cinnamon, use the following artifice. They cut all the oxen and asses and beasts of burthen that die in their land into large pieces, which they carry with them into those regions, and place near the nests: then they withdraw to a distance, and the old birds, swooping down, seize the pieces of meat and fly with them up to their nests; which, not being able to support the weight, break off and fall to the ground. Hereupon the Arabians return and collect the cinnamon, which is afterwards carried from Arabia into other countries."[74]

In Europe, cinnamon was exclusively for the rich until modern times. For example, around 300 CE, a pound of cassia cost 125 denari, the equivalent of a week's wages for a farmhand.[75] For this reason, it is excellent in magic to draw wealth or status.

Most often, cinnamon is used magically to provide a warming effect—whether to spice up a love spell or to light a fire under someone who needs to get moving. It is also an excellent offering incense, especially favored by Apollo and the dead. Nero is said to have burned a year's supply on his wife's pyre. It is also excellent for household happiness and protection. When I was little, we mixed it into apple sauce and white glue to make a sort of clay. We made small dolls from it, which we baked hard and then left around the house and yard to protect us.

Personally, I find cinnamon chips best for incense, but powdered cinnamon is okay if that's all you have. If burning powder as incense, mix in a tiny bit of water or honey to keep it from sparking. You can also just light the end of a cinnamon stick and wave it around like an incense wand.

Star Anise

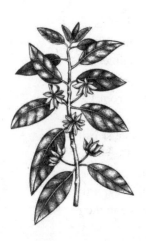

Star anise, or *Illicium verum*, is a common cooking spice, especially in Asian cuisines. It can be found in most urban grocery stores and all Asian markets. Be cautious: *Illicium anisatum* (sometimes called Japanese star anise) is toxic and shouldn't be eaten in large quantities, although it's fine for incense. If star anise seems too cheap to be believed, don't believe it; it is often adulterated with Japanese star anise. The closely related *Illicium parviflorum* is native to the southeastern United States, but rarely commercially cultivated. If it's local to you, gather it. It's good for incense, but don't cook with it.

Star anise has a long history of use in healing. Generally, for this purpose, it is brewed as tea or extracted in alcohol. Star anise tea is very effective for respiratory illnesses, including colds and flu. It's also good for upset stomachs in adults or children and as a "woman's helper": it promotes menstruation, eases PMS, aids the flow of breast milk, and increases libido in men. It can also be used in incense for all of these issues except respiratory illness. Generally, I do not recommend any incense for respiratory illness, because smoke can irritate a cough.

Magically, star anise is an excellent protection against bad luck. For this purpose, it can be strung as a garland to be hung on the front door, carried in the left pocket, or burned as incense. Star anise also aids the memory, opens the psychic senses, and promotes powerful dreaming. For dreaming, I like to steep it in milk to be drunk at bedtime, but it can also be used in a small bowl by the bedside as potpourri. Others place it under the pillow, but I don't, because the one time I tried, it broke and left little itchy bits in my bed. Be conservative when adding star anise to incense recipes; a little goes a long way.

Cardamom

Cardamom (*Elettaria cardamomum*) is among my favorite spices. It smells slightly spicy, sweet, warm, and a little woodsy or nutty. It tastes similarly, with a little bit of a green, herbal/minty undertone with a citrusy upper note. That flavor you can't identify in chai tea? That's cardamom. Personally, I love cardamom in coffee, which is common in the Middle East and Africa, but only recently seems to have caught on in the States. While they are not identical, cardamom can usually be substituted for cinnamon or vice versa in most magic. When burned as incense, cardamom is usually used as whole pods, but you can also go with just the seeds, if that's what you have. As always, avoid using ground spice if possible; it burns fast and overpowers other ingredients. If that's all you have, get it wet to slow it down a little.

Like most spices, cardamom has a long (and often bloody) history as a luxury trade good. In fact, even today, cardamom is the third most expensive spice by weight, second only to saffron and vanilla. It is excellent in wealth-drawing work, and as a rich offering for almost any spirit, but especially those of the spheres of Jupiter or Mercury. It has a long history of use in incense and perfumes, especially in men's cologne, where it adds a warm and slightly exotic flair.

Magically, cardamom's primary action is warming without being too aggressive. It is martial but has more of a "Mars at home with Venus, getting busy in the fields" vibe than "Mars on the battlefield." Cardamom is an excellent addition to aphrodisiac incense, where it both sweetens and adds a spicy kick. Cardamom can be made lusty with the addition of other spices or turned toward romance with flowers or honey. Carry seven cardamom pods in your left pocket while cruising to attract all the right sorts of attention.

Chew a little cardamom before you sweet-talk someone; it is equally good for lubricating pillow talk and boardroom negotiations. Cardamom also stimulates the right frame of mind for learning; cardamom incense is excellent for studying. If you study with cardamom incense, dab a little bit of cardamom oil on your wrists during the exam, and sniff them to stimulate your memory. Additionally, cardamom clears the mind for divination and improves the clarity of psychic channeling, although I prefer star anise for this, if you have both in stock.

Nutmeg and Mace

Nutmeg and mace are both made from the fruits of several varieties of the *Myristica* tree; nutmeg from the seed and mace from the red aril.* They are similar in smell and taste; nutmeg is slightly milder, creamier, and more delicate than mace. Mace is hotter, stronger, and more peppery and bright orange in color. For most magical purposes, they can be interchanged. In what follows, nutmeg means both nutmeg and mace.

In the United States, nutmeg is familiar. It is most often used in sweet dishes, but it's excellent in other contexts as well. Mace is more difficult to find, but is common in mixed spices, including pumpkin pie spice, many kinds of curry powders, and ras el hanout. It is also often used in ketchup. While nutmeg quickly goes stale after being ground, mace is very shelf-stable.

---

* An aril is a fleshy seed covering, such as in pomegranates.

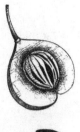

Used in the East since antiquity, nutmeg entered Europe in the Middle Ages. Until the mid-19th century, these spices were expensive imported luxury goods from Banda (a chain of Indonesian "Spice Islands"), but today they are grown throughout the tropics and readily available. That path to world distribution was a dark and terrible one. In the 1500s, the Portuguese conquered the neighboring island of Malacca, then the hub of Indonesian trade. They attempted to conquer Banda, but the Bandanese fought them off. Then the Dutch came and didn't take no for an answer. They cornered the nutmeg market by exterminating the tree on other islands. They then manipulated the European market for Indonesian spices, keeping prices artificially high at great cost in human life. In 1621, Japanese mercenaries under Dutch control slaughtered most of the political leaders of Banda and enslaved the Bandanese people. Prior to this, about fourteen thousand Bandanese lived on the island. After, about one thousand survived, nearly all of whom were enslaved laborers on nutmeg plantations. In keeping with the Dutch policy of sundering indigenous people from their land, many Bandanese were sent as slaves to other colonies, and foreign slaves were brought to Banda.

The island was "liberated" by the British in 1810, but they were more interested in saving the nutmeg trees than the Bandanese. Sufficient *Myristica* trees were transplanted to British colonies to make Banda worthless to the Dutch, who eventually gave up. Today, the Bandanese have a distinctive local culture, which combines that of the indigenous folk with those of migrants and enslaved workers brought from elsewhere in Indonesia.

The use of nutmeg as an especially rich incense is well documented. For example, in 1429, Henry VI had the streets fumigated with nutmegs for his coronation. At that time, half a kilo of nutmegs cost as much as one cow or three sheep. At the end of the Sabbath, on Saturday evening, Jewish custom dictates the smelling of rich and beautiful things; nutmeg is often used in this context.

Historically, nutmeg was used as an abortifacient, although there is not much evidence to support its effectiveness for this use. Like all abortifacient plants, nutmeg is sacred to the Witch Queens. Conversely, it is also sometimes recommended to improve fertility. It is also used as an aphrodisiac, and some clinical data supports this application. It is a vasodilator and a relaxer of smooth muscle. Like all aphrodisiacs, nutmeg is sacred to Aphrodite. In India, it is used in wedding rituals. Nutmeg is entheogenic in large quantities. Like all psychedelics, it is sacred to Hermes. Personally, I do not recommend nutmeg as an entheogen; my experience was entirely unpleasant. None of these psychedelic effects are present when used as incense. To get such a response, you would have to huff an absurd amount of incense.

Magically, nutmeg is most often used as a luck-bringer. For example, one common American folk practice is to carry a whole nutmeg in the pocket when gambling. By extension, it is also carried when in court. It can be used in love and sex-drawing magic; sprinkle nutmeg in a lover's left shoe to make them "hot to trot." Because of its association with baking, nutmeg is an excellent addition to incense designed to invoke a feeling of loving warmth, family, and home. To help sell a house, boil nutmeg in water before showings or open houses. Nutmeg can also open the psychic senses.

While I associate nutmeg primarily with the sphere of Mercury, because of its luck-bringing and entheogenic properties, many people classify it as Jupiter's because of its history. I generally recommend against the use of nutmeg for undifferentiated wealth-bringing; it is almost impossible to isolate nutmeg's history as a luxury good from its history of slavery, imperialism, and massacre. Those are not magical currents to be lightly invited into your work.

Spicebush

Spicebush (*Lindera benzoin*), which is also called "Appalachian allspice," is a flowering wild shrub native to the eastern half of the United States and Canada. It is related, but not closely, to bay laurel. It thrives in rich, wet, sunny soil. Its sweet-smelling bright-yellow flowers bloom very early and attract butterflies and moths. Spicebushes often seem to blaze a trail through the otherwise dreary wood in early spring; following that path is a good way to find magical portals. Later in the summer, it develops bright-red oval fruits, similar to hawthorn haws. These have a very distinctive spicy sweet smell similar to allspice. They are dried and used as a cooking spice and are also—along with the leaves and twigs—brewed as a delicious tea. It tastes like a citrusy, slightly more peppery allspice. In incense, you can more or less always substitute allspice for spicebush.

To find spicebush growing is a very strong sign that the surrounding land is fertile and abundant. For this reason, it is excellent in wealth and prosperity magic, just like clover. While the drupes are the part most commonly used, all parts of the plant are aromatic and can be put in incense. The fruit must be dried or stored in the freezer; the fresh berries go bad quickly. The leaves also lose their smell quickly; if using them in incense, they should be fresh. Twigs are shelf-stable.

Spicebush is used to treat a variety of reproductive complaints. Among both the Cherokee and the Rappahannock, it is known as an abortifacient.[76] Haudenosaunee healers historically used it to treat both syphilis and gonorrhea.[77] In Appalachian folk healing, it is often recommended for yeast infections. These uses hint that it is also excellent as an offering to the Witch Queens, and that has been my experience. I find spicebush to be a deeply witchy plant.

Drugs

Although almost all the ingredients we've discussed so far have pharmacological effects, the ones in this section are known primarily for their mind-altering properties. Use them sparingly and with great caution. Not all of these plants are legal in all jurisdictions.

Tobacco

Tobacco can refer to many plants of the genus *Nicotiana*, but in the United States, almost all commercially grown and sold tobacco is *Nicotiana tabacum*. *Nicotiana rustica* (Aztec tobacco) and *Nicotiana attenuata* (coyote tobacco) are also popular, but rarely commercially cultivated. In incense, any variety is fine. Undoubtedly you are familiar with the smell of burning tobacco; it is nearly unavoidable in some environments. While tobacco is very safe when used in small quantities in incense, I do not recommend it for people with sensitivities to stimulants or those who struggle with nicotine addiction.

Throughout the Americas, several types of tobacco have been grown and smoked for recreational, medicinal, and ceremonial uses for millennia. This use continues among many, many peoples including the Apache,[78] Hopi,[79] Navajo,[80] Tewa,[81] Hualapai,[82] and many others. For some, it is used in nearly every religious or magical situation imaginable. For example, among the Cahuilla, before every ritual, tobacco is smoked by both the ritual leaders and the spirit speakers, and smoke is blown to the five sacred directions to clear and sanctify the space. It is also used with weather working, agricultural magic, divination, and healing.[83]

Tobacco appears to have been cultivated at least 3,000–3,500 years ago, but it is not yet known when or where it was first domesticated.[84] In addition to its value as a plant, tobacco has also been used as a commodity currency, particularly among the indigenous peoples of eastern North America. Following the European colonization of the Americas, tobacco rapidly spread.[85] Nearly a billion people worldwide consume tobacco daily.

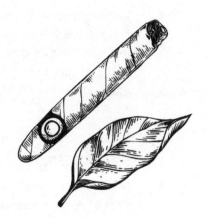

Because I grew up in tobacco country, I associate it very strongly with the Land and use it primarily in offering blends for nature spirits. However, it is also excellent as an offering for the dead. When I need to make an unexpected offering or work in a graveyard with the restless dead unprepared, I often borrow a cigarette from someone and use it as an incense stick. Cigarettes are also a common graveside offering, along with dimes and clean water. Among the Cahuilla people, mourners at a funeral are strongly encouraged to smoke tobacco, because the smoke helps to concentrate their powerful remembrance, helping the dead on their journey along the Long Road.[86]

Tobacco can be spread across a rival's doorway as a malefic trick. In other contexts, tobacco can be protective. The Kawaiisu throw tobacco, along with lime, in their campfires to ward off malicious spirits.[87] In many cultures, small pouches of tobacco are hung around the belly of a pregnant person or the neck of an infant to ward off evil spirits. However, I do *not* recommend this practice, because of the likelihood of the baby sucking on it.

In many types of traditional South American trance healing, tobacco smoke is blown from the healer's mouth onto the patient's body to facilitate the exchange of magical energy; mugwort, marijuana, and many other plants can also be smoked and used in this way. Similarly, tobacco smoke can be used to bless and empower poppets and other ritual items. I find tobacco especially effective for martial magic. Because modern commercial tobacco is largely bred and grown by immoral death merchants, I generally do not recommend using it in healing magic.

As a magical drug, tobacco is primarily a stimulant and functions to produce visions and aid in trance magic and vision quests. In addition to its nearly ubiquitous indigenous use across the Americas, tobacco has been employed for hundreds of years for this purpose all around the globe, particularly among Arab and Russian traditional trance healers. Nicotine and other stimulants do not agree with me, so I do not have much experience of this state. Personally, I would not use commercially grown tobacco for this purpose; it is too spiritually polluted by human greed to be a reliable teacher and has long been bred to be even more addictive than wild tobacco.

Marijuana

Marijuana (*Cannabis sativa*) is a flowering plant likely indigenous to the Central Asia subcontinent.[88] It has been used in incense for as long as humans have been recording such matters, and solid archaeological evidence indicates it has been prized by humans in Asia almost as long as there have been humans in Asia.[89] Although it is unclear whether it was present in the Americas before European colonization, it has unquestionably been extensively cultivated everywhere else on Earth for many, many millennia and is in widespread cultivation in the Americas since the earliest days of European colonization. In the modern day, cannabis has been so completely domesticated that most commercial strains cannot reproduce by themselves.

The most important thing to remember, when reconstructing antique recipes that contain marijuana, is that modern marijuana is *much, much, much* more powerful a drug than the marijuana called for in those recipes. According to some studies, modern marijuana as of 2020 has been bred to contain almost ten times as much THC as it did just twenty years ago.[90] Compared to the cannabis of our ancestors, modern marijuana is a miracle. Quantities need to be dramatically reduced when adapting historical recipes containing marijuana. For medical-strength strains, I generally recommend one part modern marijuana for every fifteen parts called for in a premodern recipe. In the recipes included in this book, which obviously should only be used in jurisdictions where it is legal to do so, I have already made that conversion.

Historically, human-cultivated marijuana smoke has been used magically and spiritually for at least 2,500 years.[91] Archaeological evidence at a cemetery in the Pamir Plateau (modern Tajikistan) indicates cannabis unusually high in THC was smoked in braziers.[92] Their location in a cemetery is very strong evidence for their use in ritual or as an offering to the dead. Residue from the combustion of naturally occurring cannabis has been found on the altars at Tel Arad temple in the Negev Desert, where it was burned with frankincense and several other ingredients.[93]

The Scythians, a Bronze Age people of Central Asia, used it as part of their hero/ancestor cult. According to Herodotus, after the death of a king or hero, the people would build small hot-boxing tents in which "having taken some seed of this hemp, they creep under the cloths and put the seeds on the red-hot stones; but this being put on smokes, and produces such a steam, that no Grecian vapour-bath would surpass it. The Scythians, transported by the vapour, shout aloud."[94]

In incense, marijuana's effects are not as potent as when smoked, both because of the small quantities used and also because it diffuses into the air. In incense, marijuana is almost always used to open the psychic senses and promote spirit manifestation. It can generally be substituted with a mixture of mugwort and amanita mushrooms or wormwood and damiana.

Amanita Mushrooms

Fly agaric (*Amanita muscaria*) is the most famous of the toadstool mushrooms. If you imagine a fairy mushroom, red with white spots, you're probably picturing *Amanita muscaria*. Although it is native only in the forests of the Northern Hemisphere, it now grows worldwide, wherever pine trees do. Without careful preparation, *Amanita muscaria* is toxic to ingest, but is safe in incense.

Amanita mushrooms have a long history of both ritual and recreational use among peoples of the Arctic Circle and their slightly southern neighbors. It is particularly well documented among the Sami people of northern Scandinavia and Uralic-speaking peoples of Siberia and the Russian Far East. It is also known to be used ritually in Lithuania, Afghanistan, and among the Ojibwe nation in Canada. In all of these cases, it appears to be used as a trance aid primarily, but not exclusively by trained spirit-workers or those in ritual with them.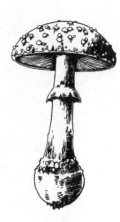

In incense, any type of dried mushroom adds a delicate earthy "forest floor" and is excellent for work connected to the Land, the life-death-decay-life cycle, and the chthonic gods. Amanita is good for all of these purposes, and particularly excellent for work with the Good Neighbors. When burned, it has a mild mind-expanding action that is subtler and more visceral than marijuana. The effect from inhaling smoke is very subtle compared to ingestion, but it is noticeable, especially if the incense is huffed or smoked. Experiment carefully.

Non-Plant Materials

MANY UNEXPECTED ingredients can be added to incense to produce magical effects. For the most part, these fall into two broad categories: combustible and inert. Combustible materials are those that will be impacted by burning. This includes all the ingredients we've spoken about so far, but also lots of other non-plant materials. I'll speak about a few of my favorites below, but you can also experiment with your own. It is very important to test *outside* in open air how materials react to burning before adding them to incense; many things you wouldn't expect to do so can spark, explode, or produce really noxious or even poisonous smoke.

Honey

As you'll see once we proceed to the recipes, I love using honey in incense. Its stickiness binds the other ingredients together, and it gives huge clouds of thick sweet, slightly floral smoke, perfect to scry or evoke into. You can try adding honey to almost any mixture to increase the smoke volume. Similarly, if you want less smoke, take out the honey.

Honey is a powerful healing ally. In particular, it is excellent for coughs and as balm on burns, abrasions, or other small skin wounds, like new tattoos. Honey is a very common offering, particularly favored by gods of cold places. It is also a special favorite of Hekate, Min (an Egyptian fertility god), and Zeus. In his infancy, Zeus was fed honey by the nymph Melissa and milk from the divine nanny goat Amalthea. In Judaism, honey and apples are eaten at the New Year to ensure sweetness in the coming year. I have been taught that this is because they represent two different kinds of sweetness. The apples represent expected sweetness. We all know fruits are sweet. Honey, on the other hand, is regurgitated by stinging insects and so its sweetness is an unexpected delight.

The bee was the symbol of Lower Egypt, that is the Nile Delta in the north. Among the ancient Greeks, bees symbolized industry and hard work, just as they do in our own culture. However, they were also very closely associated with prophecy, particularly at the oracle of Apollo at Delphi and that of Trophonios (Τροφώνιος) in Lebadeia. There is a legend that says that the first temple at Delphi was made of bay laurel leaves and the second was built by bees. One way to understand this is to say that the wealth and power of Delphi was founded on their bay and honey trade.

Magically, honey can be used in several ways. The first is that local honey, which is basically the distilled essence of all the flowers in a neighborhood, is an *excellent* ingredient to use when working with your local land spirits. Similarly, honey from other locations can be used to call on the powers of those places. If you travel to places that hold power, try to bring some local honey home with you. Most commonly, honey is used as a magical sweetener, particularly in a type of work called a honey pot.

THE HONEY POT

Honey pots are a traditional kind of sweetening work, that is, work intended to make the target "sweet" on you. They can be used as love spells, but are more often used to make a relative, neighbor, or boss be nicer to you. The version I teach below is strongly informed by Hoodoo, a tradition of African American folk magic from the American South, with roots in the practices of enslaved Africans, indigenous Americans, and European colonists. However, very similar methods are known in many cultures and broadly called sweetening spells. In the example below, I'll be sweetening a whole family/household on each other. This is a common tactic to reduce tension and drama in a home. I'm doing it with honey, but the spell can be done in an almost identical way with sugar or any other sweetener.

YOU WILL NEED:

A jar of honey

A small empty jar that is not shaped like a bear

Herbs/spices that support your intent and are deliciously sweet. Vanilla or
rose are good for love. Cinnamon is homey. A hint of black pepper can
spice things up. And so on.

Paper and pen

Photos and names of the targets

A plate

A gold-colored coin

A tea light

About half an hour of crafting time and half an hour of suspended
disbelief. These need not be contiguous.

WHAT TO DO:

♦ Begin by writing a short description of what you want. In this
example, my intent is *"All who eat of this honey are linked by
bonds of love, friendship, and hospitality."*

♦ Shorten your intent to a few words. *"Love, Friendship,
Hospitality."*

♦ Shorten that into a single "barbarous name" for the working. I generally do this by mushing together the sounds until it seems right;
others make anagrams or use other word play. You can apply any
method that seems right to you. In this case, I settled on *"Lofrenospy,"* which I pronounce *"loh-FREN-ahs-pee."*

♦ On the paper, write the names of your targets, three times each.

♦ Turn the paper ninety degrees and write your barbarous name over
them nine times.

♦ Roll this paper up, and put it in the empty jar, along with photos of
the targets.

♦ If using herbs or other combustibles, add them to the jar now.

♦ Put the jar on a plate.

- Enter into magical time, space, and consciousness by any method.

- Slowly, sloooooowwwly pour honey into the jar. While you do so, chant your barbarous name.

- Watch the honey seep into the contents of the jar. Feel the jar awaken to life.

- Keep chanting and pouring until the jar slightly overflows onto the plate.

- Speak directly from your heart to the jar, addressing it by name. Introduce yourself. Butter it up. Tell it why you have awakened it. Make your specific request. Thank it for helping you. In our example, I might say, *"I greet you, Lofrenospy. I am Sara. I, Sara, have awakened you, Lofrenospy, to help me spread love, friendship, and hospitality. Oh, Lofrenospy, sweet and delicious one, alchemical essence of the flowers and herbs, golden nectar of magic, I ask you to help me! Let all who eat of this honey be linked by bonds of love, friendship, and hospitality. In thanks I give you this coin."*

- Drop the coin in the jar.

- Close the jar and put the candle on top of (or in front of) the jar. Light it.

- Exit magical space, time, and consciousness.

- After the candle burns down, open the jar and add a small amount of the enchanted honey back into your regular eating honey to "infect" all who taste it with the spell. You can repeat this every time you open a new jar of eating honey. Add a new coin to the jar every you take out a sample.

Making baked goods with the enchanted honey and taking them to work—or wherever—is a classic tactic in sweetening magic.

Scrolls

Small petition scrolls, sigils, or other papers can always be added to incense. Keep them as small as possible. Be cautious; paper produces a lot of smoke and can set off smoke detectors. If making incense in large quantities to store for future use, petition papers, etc., can be placed inside the container with the incense during storage to empower both scroll and incense.

Animal Parts

I rarely use animal parts in my incense, but they are a common feature of many, many traditional recipes. Hair from black dogs is a common ingredient in malefic magic, particularly for making lovers or partners fight or split up. Hair from black cats is often called for in similar works, although it can also be used to bring luck, especially for gambling. Many types of feathers are common in magic, and this is the only animal part I regularly use. All feathers are good for work with the element of Air, but the individual properties depend on the character of the bird they came from. For example, crow feathers are excellent in malefica, while goose feathers are good for abundance work. To use feathers, cut off the barbs (the soft part) with scissors. Only use 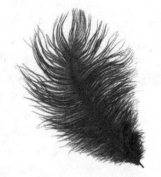 a little; they smell bad when burned. Snakeskin is an excellent addition to many magical incenses, including any involving serpentine spirits, and also many types of malefica. Like most animal parts, it has an unpleasant smell. Use only a little bit.

Human Parts

With the exception of scrolls, the non-plant combustible material I most often add to incense is human body parts: hair, fingernails, blood, and sexual fluids, for example. These are usually to link the magic to the person I'm trying to affect. You can also use other people's sexual fluids to impact their sexual performance, either to invigorate or wilt. Blood can be added to tie an incense directly to your physical body; this is sometimes appropriate for healing magic. Blood can also be used as bait in incense to attract infernal or otherwise vampiric spirits. In general, that is not a practice appropriate to beginners. Materials like hair or nails can also be added to aggressive magic to target a victim. They stink when burned.

Dirt

Dirt from various locations can also be added, to bring to an incense mixture the power of the location where it was gathered. This is particularly relevant when the target of the magic is, itself, a location, such as in spells to sell a house or get a job at a specific office. Dirt from sacred sites is excellent. So is dirt from crossroads, used for magic related to travel or communication. I also like dirt from the grave sites of people relevant to the work at hand. Some people recommend gathering dirt from graves of unknown people based on their profession (such as a police officer's grave for protection), but I do not advise that, because you never really know on whom you're calling. However, I am strongly in favor of using dirt from the graves of ancestors, loved ones, or famous people whose biography you know. You can add a tiny pinch to any loose incense, but I more often use it on top of the heat sink—or as a heat sink, if I have enough of it—under the charcoal. For the most part, dirt doesn't burn, but it often has dried leaves and such mixed in which might. As always, do a test burn.

Coins

My favorite noncombustible materials are coins. I do not so much add them to the incense as I use them for a base. Sometimes, I fill a bowl with them, and put the charcoal on top. Sometimes, I put a single coin on top of the charcoal and place the incense on top of that. This provides for a slower burn for the incense and also leaves you with a coin imbued with the magical force of the incense.

Coin magic is a deep and rich subject I cannot possibly do justice to here, and doubtless you will find your own uses as you experiment. One thing I frequently do is awaken the person, animals, or scenes on them, most often for political magic. Additionally, I use U.S. coins as follows in the chart on page 97:

Pennies	Venus, love, romance, friendship. Wheat pennies are good for "happy home" magic. Carry seven pennies in your left pocket to draw romance to you.
Nickels	Mars, strength, endurance, aggressive and defensive magic. Carry five nickels in your right pocket to help you be assertive.
Dimes	Mercury, the dead, luck. So-called "Mercury dimes" or "Winged Liberty dimes" are especially good for this. Leave a dime on a grave each time you visit, but especially if you take anything. Among my paternal family, finding a dime on the ground is considered a sign from our ancestors, telling us that they are still with us.
Quarters	Now that there are so many kinds of quarters, I use them as talismans for many purposes, based on the image on the reverse side. The eagle-backed ones are excellent for Jupiter.
Gold dollars	I use these for solar and healing work, but primarily for prosperity-drawing magic. These also come in many varieties, which can be used based on their design.

Part Three

Recipes

Incense to Set a Scene

IF YOU'VE READ through the previous chapters, you've come to know a whole slew of amazing incense ingredients, most of which can be burned on their own. However, the fun of incense making comes in combining ingredients together to make more complicated smells. In this part, you'll learn many of my favorite incense recipes, but, more importantly, you'll start to learn how to adapt, experiment, and improvise your own recipes for any kind of occasion, offering, or spell.

The simplest, but in many ways the most difficult, method to develop a recipe for incense is to determine the vibe you want to impart to a space as an actual setting, with rich cinematic details, including imagining what that place smells like. The easiest way to learn to do this is to pay careful attention to the smells of places you encounter. Throughout your day, smell things you come across: plants, foods, soaps, people,* and rooms. Describe those smells to yourself, comparing them to the scents you've learned. If you've been working your way through the book so far, you should have a good mental library of scent memories to compare things to, to help you identify smells. Remember that the goal isn't to exactly recreate smells, but rather to transport the smeller to other places. Pick some favorite mythic or fictional settings and imagine what they smell like. Where do you wish you were right now? What sort of mood do you want to set?

---

*   Obviously, I am not encouraging you to sniff people like a crazy stalker.

Bacchic Revel

Imagine yourself in a wild meadow, just before the sun slips below the horizon. Warm Mediterranean breezes caress your barely clad body. Welcome to the Witch's Sabbat and the Great Bacchanal. The rite has not yet begun, but revelers, human and otherwise, have gathered, and tension hangs on the wind. Suddenly, drums begin to throb in the air . . .

This is the incense I burn when I throw parties. It imbues the space with an aura of fun, passion, creativity, and safety while taking the edge off any anxiety, hostility, or drama, all while covering a fair bit of smoke and body odor. It is also nice as an offering to Bacchus.

> 2 parts frankincense or another resin to bring light, purity, and
>   good vibes
> 2 parts damiana to put everyone in the mood to have a good time
> 1 part catnip to keep everything chill and drama-free
> 1 part cinnamon to bring the warmth of conviviality
> 1 part ground raisins soaked in wine to bind everyone together in
>   sweetness and mirth

The Isles of Witches

This is the incense I burn when I cannot handle living in the loud, dirty, crowded city for a single minute more. When I want to retreat to a magical island where no one can find me, this is the incense I turn to. It comes in two versions, Avalon and Aeaea, which could equally well have been called "Cool" and "Warm." I most often burn them cross-seasonally. When it's cold out, I want to be on sunny Aeaea, and in the brutal summer heat I long for cool, green Avalon.

VERSION ONE: AVALON

Sometimes, the world is loud and fast and too, too bright. Sometimes, I want to rest, dream, and just be in someplace cool, peaceful, and silvery sylvan green. The place I imagine at those times is Avalon, the magical island home of Morgana le Fey and the burial place of King Arthur. The full moon fights to shine through a heavy gray rain, but I'm snuggled safe behind heavy stone walls, basking at a crackling pine fire. Apples and herbs hang from the rafters, drying. My mind cools and calms, the stress of the day left behind, and I feel myself opening to restorative relaxation, instructive dreams, and deep healing.

The oldest known use of the name "Avalon" is in the 1136 CE *Historia Regum Britanniae*, a brilliant piece of historical fiction recounting the story of Britain from the time of its founding by Trojan refugees until the conquest of the Anglo-Saxons. In the book, the author describes Avalon (which means "Apple-land") as the origin of King Arthur's legendary sword Excalibur. In a later work, *Vita Merlini* ("The Life of Merlin"), Geoffrey of Monmouth tells of a council of nine sisters, led by the enchantress Morgan, who rule over the island, which is said to be "where the ladies are who follow all the enchantments of the world." Many people, including the 12th-century commentator Gerald of Wales, equate Avalon with the Tor of Glastonbury, which was an island before the surrounding swamps were drained.

In addition to setting a scene, this incense is also excellent as a light aid to trance work or as an offering to the Good Neighbors or Morgana le Fey, a splendid teacher of witchcraft. But, as I said, I most often use this incense with no intent past creating a calm, sacred, magical mood. This incense can also be used as a bath, if you omit the pine resin. Use a cloth bag; it will make a mess in the bathtub otherwise.

2 parts pine resin to capture the crackling fire

4 parts mugwort to evoke the herbs that hang from the rafters, as is

1 part vervain

2 parts dried apples for the Isle of Apples

2 parts hyssop for the meadows wavering in the breeze

1 part hawthorn berries (While the Glastonbury Thorn rarely produces
    haws, all hawthorn is emblematic of both Glastonbury and Avalon.)

VERSION TWO: AEAEA

Sometimes, the world is heavy, oppressive, and too, too dark. Sometimes, I want to rest, dream, and just be in someplace warm, lush, and dappled with golden light. The place I imagine at these times is Aeaea, the mythic island where Odysseus encountered the great witch Circe, daughter of Helios, fosterling of Hekate. The sun is setting over the Mediterranean, and the ever-dulcet west wind caresses my hair. I'm standing at the window of a tower in a shining white marble palace, a pet lioness asleep at my feet. Herbs and dates hang drying in my pharmacy, and pine crackles in the brazier. My mind relaxes and unfolds, blossoming like a flower in the sun, opening to inspiration, revelation, and healing.

The oldest known reference to Aeaea (Αἰαία) is in Homer's *Odyssey*, a brilliant adventure tale telling the story of Odysseus, a hero of the Trojan War, trying to find his way home while under the curse of the sea god Poseidon. In the *Odyssey*, we are told that when Odysseus arrives there, Aeaea is ruled by a witch-queen, Circe. At first, Circe and Odysseus are enemies, but they soon become lovers. Eventually, Odysseus leaves to continue his journey, after Circe teaches him how to descend into the Underworld to seek wisdom from the dead. Homer does not give details as to its location, except to place it in the Eastern Mediterranean. In the *Argonautica*, Jason and Medea come to Aeaea from Colchis, hoping for healing and absolution from Circe. There, its location is described with more precision: south of Elba, within sight of the shores of western Italy.

Both works describe a community of women, led by Circe, who live together and practice witchcraft on the island, and that is the Aeaea I imagine, which exists in a time and space apart from our world, afloat in the great River Okeanos, who encircles both our World and the Other Place. I believe it to be a great center of teaching, where the sisterhood of witches that begins with Gaia, Phoebe, and Hekate and continues through Circe, Morgana, Hildegard, and many others continues to learn and to teach. I have been there in my dreams, and I encourage you to seek it out as well.

2 parts Chios mastic for the warm Mediterranean sun

3 parts mugwort for the drying herbs, along with . . .

2 parts dittany of Crete

1 part orange peel for clarity and joy

1 part cinnamon for warmth

1 part raisins for the sweetness of the wine

Fortress of Solitude

Far from any human habitation, the wind whistles across the ice-numbed tundra. Spires of ice reach toward the sky, and beyond them, the great glacier glowers, an endless wall of ice. In the wall of ice hangs a golden door that opens only for me. A shower of ice crystals sprinkles down, glittering in the sun, as the door swings open. It clangs into place behind me, and I know that I am utterly and completely alone. No one can see me here. What happens in the Fortress of Solitude stays in the Fortress of Solitude.

> 1 part sandalwood for the soft quiet of the snow
>
> 1 part lemon peel for the bright sparkling ice
>
> 2 parts juniper needles for the sharp, piercing spires
>
> 1 part resin for the glowing golden door

Hobbit Hole

"Not a nasty, dirty, wet hole, filled with the ends of worms and an oozy smell, nor yet a dry, bare, sandy hole with nothing in it to sit down on or to eat: it was a hobbit-hole, and that means comfort."[95] This is my go-to kitchen blend and what's burning in my house most of the time. It creates a warm, welcome, convivial atmosphere ready for impromptu get-togethers with friends. It's also great at family gatherings.

> 3 parts pine resin for warmth and joy
>
> 3 parts kitchen sage for peace
>
> 1 part cinnamon for coziness
>
> 1 part thyme for adventure
>
> Honey to bind it with sweetness

Cybermagic MakerSpace

This is the incense I turn to when I want to make believe that I'm in a super futuristic magical maker-space. It's where I build my time machines and spaceships, and also what I burn in my real-world workshop. I used to burn it in my classroom when I was a teacher. It's also good as an offering for spirits of technology or while learning math and science.

> 3 parts frankincense to bring solar power
>
> 2 parts apples for the fruit of knowledge and the Great Teacher
>
> 1 part black pepper for a slightly acrid electrical tang
>
> 2 parts peppermint to add a sleek and clean futuristic feeling and to stimulate the mind

The Spa of the Nymphs

Imagine a spa, secluded in a deep forest, far from any prying eyes. Cool rain pitter-patters down onto the cedar roof, while the waters of the hot spring bubble up all around you. An herbal salve tingles on your skin, and the fire pops and hisses, filling the sauna with warm, fragrant steam. Your body relaxes, and you can finally feel yourself think. Dryads massage you with scented oils and bring you frothy drinks. A gaggle of river nymphs giggle and wiggle their toes in the mud, trading idle gossip. Have you heard what Artemis did to that creep they caught peeping last week? I often burn this incense while I'm in the bathtub, and it can also be used as a sachet in the bath (leave out the resin) or compounded as an oil.

> 4 parts cedar
>
> 2 parts resin
>
> 2 parts mint
>
> 1 part sage
>
> 1 part damiana
>
> 1 part dittany of Crete
>
> 1 part rose
>
> 1 part citrus peel

The Great Library

Bright golden sun shines in through leaded windows, illuminating the tables of the Great Library. Against every wall, shelves stretch up to the arches far above, piled high with scrolls, manuscripts, books, disks, and futuristic storage devices. People, human and otherwise, from a hundred different cultures work quietly beside each other, occasionally huddling together to whisper excitedly. Elders sit by the fire, drinking tea and playing four-dimensional chess. In the outer courtyard of the Musaeum, a priestess sings while she lights incense. The air smells like old books, magic, and inspiration.

> 3 parts mixed resins
>
> 2 parts chai tea
>
> 1 part vanilla
>
> 1 part tobacco (optional)
>
> 1 part clover flower

This incense is also appropriate as an offering to Hypatia, Thoth, or the librarian or scribal spirit of your choice. Experiment with different kinds of tea for different "branch libraries."

The Holy Mountain of the Monks

As I mentioned in the introduction, the Greek monastic community on Mount Athos, famed for its incense, has forbidden women for over a thousand years. As you might imagine, that makes me desperately want to go! This incense is not designed to replicate the incenses manufactured on Mount Athos, but rather it is what I imagine the island itself smells like. It is excellent for meditation or personal spiritual work. I often burn this when I'm writing. It layers a typical Greek Orthodox church incense over a base of Greek mountain herbs and trees.

> 6 parts frankincense
>
> 4 parts myrrh
>
> 1 part mastic
>
> 2 parts rose
>
> 4 parts cedarwood
>
> 2 parts juniper needles
>
> 1 part dittany of Crete
>
> 1 part rosemary
>
> Honey to bind

Romance Novel

This incense was inspired by the Twitter account @RomanceSmells, which catalogs romance novels' descriptions of how men smell. While it can be used in love or sex magic, it's intended as an atmospheric blend for the bedroom, for when we single ladies or fellows or folx want to light some candles and show ourselves a good time. I strongly encourage you to develop your own signature blends. I've provided a few examples for inspiration. These formulas can also be compounded as perfume oils.

BASE RECIPE

> 2 parts cedarwood
>
> 3 parts juniper needles
>
> 1 part damiana
>
> 1 part tobacco
>
> 1 part myrrh

DEMON LOVER

> Replace the cedar with sandalwood, increase the myrrh, and add a little cardamom.

TACITURN WEREWOLF

> Replace the damiana with amanita and the tobacco with mugwort.

IO PAN

> Replace the tobacco with patchouli and add some dried berries.

DREAMY POET

> Double the tobacco and add one part bay leaves.

MOODY DRUMMER

> Add one part cloves and one part coffee beans.

FARM BOY

> Change the myrrh to pine, drop the tobacco, and add one part lemongrass.

Change the cedar to pine, the myrrh to mastic, and add one part tarragon.

The House of Healing

Nestled into the Northern Woods, the home of Grandmother Winter is where I want to be when I'm sick. Outside the window, I can hear the rain—soft and cool and calm. Cool, crisp white linen sheets and soft gray blankets cocoon me. Nourishing soup bubbles over a crackling fire. A tingling salve opens my congested chest. There's nowhere better to convalesce than here, where I am safe and cared for.

> 1 part cedarwood for the Great Forest
>
> 2 parts juniper (or other needles) for the smell of the Northern Woods
>
> 4 parts mugwort (or another artemisia) to evoke the primary smell of the house of healing (It grows in huge hedges around the garden.)
>
> 3 parts pine (or another resin) to capture the warmth and comfort of the fireplace
>
> 1 part thyme for the smell of healing soup bubbling on the fireplace, as is . . .
>
> 1 part kitchen sage to gently cleanse and bring peace while it heals
>
> 1 part elderberries for their powerful healing magic and the favor of Grandmother Winter

I encourage you to seek the House of Healing, deep in the Northern Woods, in your own dreams and journeys. Burn this incense in your bedroom when you're sick, both to help refresh the space and to aid you in finding your way. If you have a cough, burn the incense in the empty room and allow the smoke to settle before entering. Perhaps take a hot bath while it smokes. Once you're in bed, say the following charm to incubate a dream of the House of Healing.

One, two, three gates north I go.

Over the river and through the woods I go.

Tap, tap, tap goes Woodpecker's nose.

Follow him deeper, past the yews, past the rose.

Over the river and through the woods I go.

Past the well, and past the dell, and past the apple grove.

Follow my nose, the smoke is the road,

Smell the herbs and the all-healing smoke.

Over the river and through the woods I go.

Basic Offering Incenses

PERHAPS AS AN extension of its uses as medicine and sensual delight, incense has a long and storied history of use as an offering to the Divine in almost every culture. Incense's particular value as an offering rests on several foundations:

- It covers the sometimes unpleasant smells of other kinds of burnt offerings.

- It comes in many varieties and so is highly customizable.

- It is value-dense, which makes it an in-demand trade good and, by extension, a good thing to trade the spirits for wishes granted.

- The smoke travels upward toward the heavens and diffuses outward, which is important symbolically, and also makes it a nice choice for large public rituals with an audience; you can see and smell a large incense offering, even from the cheap seats.

My personal offering practices are broadly based on biblical offerings. The Hebrew word for an offering is קָרְבָּן (korban), which means something like "be near to" or "draw close." The same word can also mean "a vow." I make many kinds of offerings for many reasons. The types below are not intended as strict categories, but rather broad themes intended only to inspire you to develop your own practices.

The first type of offering I make is the maintenance offering. This is just like feeding a pet or watering a plant. Offerings give spirits a foothold in the physical world. This is especially beneficial for less-powerful and less-communicatory spirits. For the most part, I offer water, candles, and incense as maintenance offerings. For a denser maintenance offering, for spirits with little power of their own, I add grains, a whole egg in the shell, oil, and honey.

Next are thanksgiving offerings. When a spirit has really come through for me, either by producing something I specifically asked for or arranging something I didn't even know I wanted, I make an extra offering. Incense is a nice thanksgiving offering, but I like to combine it with something fancier. Usually, this is a whole raw egg cracked into a glass of whole milk, but sometimes it's something else I know they'll like or something negotiated between us previously as payment for the requested service.

During ritual, especially with new spirits, I make preliminary offerings as bait to convince them to come to meet me. When I do something to offend a spirit, I make a sin offering. Just as it does with humans, a proper apology to a spirit consists of three parts: an admission of wrongdoing, an expression of regret, and an attempt at restitution. If you really messed up, as with humans, baked goods rarely go amiss.

Finally, the type of offering most central to my practice, which I was surprised to discover is unusual, is hospitality offerings. In my kitchen, I have a special altar I call the "wet egg," at which I dispense offerings to all spirits. I am not feeding them because I want something from them or because I think I owe them something. I'm feeding them because they are hungry and I am not. I burn many types of incense at this altar, usually just a pinch of whatever I'm making that day.

In this chapter, you'll learn basic offering incenses for many types of spirits. However, it is important to keep in mind that these types are largely a matter of human linguistic convenience. In practice, the type to which a spirit is assigned is as much about the language and culture of the human being they are in relationship with, and the nature and structure of that relationship, as it is an essential property of the spirit. *Angel*, for example, means "messenger"; it's a job description, not a species. As incarnate beings, we are used to thinking of individual persons as having very clear boundaries between them. Those boundaries are the very essence of bodies. And yet, even for us embodied folk, there are moments of ecstatic intimacy where we know that the line between *I* and *Thou* is a tenuous veil.

For creatures without bodies, these boundaries are far more ephemeral and diffuse. Here, as everywhere, we simplify to learn. Do not mistake the map for the terrain.

The cosmological model in which I most frequently work magic, the so-called "Three Worlds cosmology," is widely shared across many cultures. I have chosen it for this book only as one example and as a simple way to organize the types of spirits and offerings we'll be talking about. Before we move on to recipes for offering incenses, we'll take a brief tour of the three. We'll begin in the so-called Middle World, which can also be called Here or Home or Earth, and which some people think of as the "Real World." In addition to humans and other living creatures, it is populated primarily by nature spirits.

From Here, there are two directions to go. You can go up to the Upper World (or Heavens) or down to the Underworld. The Upper World is often understood as a series of spheres surrounding the Earth. The first (lowest) heaven is more or less the same place as Here; it runs from the surface of the Earth up to the outer edges of the atmosphere. We live at the very bottom of the lowest heaven, although we often think of ourselves as living "on" Earth. We do not. We are creatures of the lower sky. This region is sometimes called the sublunary sphere by Western magicians.

Above this are the seven planetary spheres: Moon, Mercury, Venus, Sun, Mars, Jupiter, and Saturn. In this context, *planet* does not mean "large, dense, nonluminous body orbiting a star"; it means "object that wanders the heavens." Above the planetary spheres are the sphere of the fixed stars and then a variety of far celestial realms. The Heavens are inhabited by many types of spirits, including angels, so-called intelligences, most gods and other mythological creatures, planetary and stellar spirits, and several other types of beings.

Finally, there is the Underworld, which is below Here. There is a significant amount of cultural agreement about the denizens and geography of the Underworld, far more so than about the Heavens or the Middle World. I suspect this is because, when we go up from where we are, we can each get to a different place, but if you go far enough down anywhere on Earth, we're all headed to the same place. That is the special nature of downness. It is distinct from upness because of gravity; down is down because of the mass of the Earth. Here on our round planet, all "downs" go the same place: first to the center of the Earth, and then "further down" into the same Underworld. That, I believe, is why most people have very similar experiences when traveling to the Underworld.

The World Tree

The World Tree is a cosmological phenomenon described by many, many cultures all over the world. It is a huge tree that serves as an axis mundi, connecting the many worlds. Its leaves are in the Heavens and its roots in the Underworld. Different cultures describe the World Tree's myth and function similarly, although it presents as many different species of tree. In fact, there is not one singular World Tree; rather all trees, to one extent or another, participate in the Great World Tree.

There are huge "public" world trees, which are shared by large numbers of people, such as Yggdrasil, the Norse World Tree. However, there are also many, many other World Trees. In fact, each person has their own personal World Tree, which is closely allied with their spine. It is along this personal World Tree that we travel between the worlds.

Imagine a tree whose roots are in the Underworld and whose leaves are in the Heavens. There is probably a hollow opening of some sort that will function like a door. If you have a good visual imagination, you may be picturing it clearly already. If so, flip through some pictures of tree species online until you can identify what type of tree it is. Try working with that species as your World Tree, and try burning its wood as incense.

If you can't see it clearly, that's okay too. Some people, including me, just don't have strong visual imaginations. If this is the case for you as well, you can imagine your tree by name instead of image. However, discovering a tree's name is harder, so try to manage a picture if you can. Alternatively, you may use a public world tree until you find your own. If you would like to try to determine what sort of tree your World Tree is, try answering the following questions as quickly as you can. Try not to think about the answers before responding. Don't decide. Don't determine. Just guess. Some of these questions may or may not apply to you; they are just to jog your intuition. You'll know when you find the right one, as it will sort of click and just feel right. Experiment with several types of trees until you find one—or more—that works for you.

- Did you have a tree house as a kid? What kind of tree was it?

- When you were a child, which tree was your friend?

- Is there a particular tree under which you pour out offerings? What kind of tree is it?

- What kind(s) of trees grow on land you tend?

- Imagine the white rabbit from *Alice in Wonderland*. When, as a child, you imagined following him as he ducked into the roots of a tree, what kind of tree was it?

- Imagine Winnie the Pooh's Hundred Acre Wood. Remember how each character lives in a tree house? When you imagined living in the Wood, what kind of tree was your house?

- Imagine shape-shifting into a tree. What kind of tree are you?

- Imagine the Great Tree whom all trees worship. Describe it.

- When your very first human incarnation died, what sort of tree grew on your grave?

WORLD TREE OFFERING INCENSE

For our first recipe, we have this very simple incense. It is excellent for all kinds of magic, especially that work called hedge riding or trance journeying and as a general offering for all spirits of all the worlds. The World Tree can also help distribute your offerings to creatures and spirits of all three worlds. This incense is ideal for that purpose.

The first three ingredients represent the three worlds of most traditional animist cosmologies, and the last, your personal World Tree(s). If you keep only one offering incense in stock to give to everyone, this is the one I would recommend. After the recipe, we'll discuss several variations. This incense is very mildly entheogenic, but the effect is too small to notice unless you lean directly into the smoke and huff a lot of it.

INGREDIENTS

3 parts resin (Native resin is best for this, but any resin is fine.)

3 parts mugwort or another artemisia (Local is best.)

3 parts amanita mushrooms

1 part wood from your personal World Tree

Honey to bind

When making magical incenses or other magic potions, many people like to awaken each ingredient to its magical potential before beginning. This is a simple process. After entering into magical time, space, and consciousness, speak to each ingredient, reminding it that it was once alive, calling it by its names of power, and helping it to remember the powers of its spirit, highlighting those that are relevant to the work at hand. In this and the other early recipes, I'll give you specific hymns to each ingredient you can use, but as the book progresses, I'll wean you off of my words and help you learn to craft your own. Here are some examples:

Eastern White Pine, golden tears of the sacred tree, I awaken you to yourself and to your many powers. Tree of Peace, great one, you reach up, up, up for the heavens and the shining warmth of the sun. You are sunshine made material and the love of the heavens incarnate. Pine, son of the sun and daughter of the heavens, you are the highest of the high. Bless this incense with your celestial fires, and warm the heart of all who breathe you in. Bring the heavens down to me and carry my wishes up in your smoke.

Mugwort, sacred plant of the Divine Huntress, you are the very essence of the greenling wood. You bring peace and dreams. You protect from every ill and safeguard the soul against possession. You warm the heart and bring lightness to the soul. Remember, Mugwort, what you made known, what you arranged at the Great Proclamation. You were called Una, the oldest of herbs; you have power against three and against thirty; you have power against poison and against infection; you have power against the loathsome foe roving through the land. Mugwort, blessed daughter of the Middle World, bless this incense with your green magic, and bring healing and insight to all who breathe you in. Bring all the world here to me, and carry my wishes out in your smoke.

Amanita, red-spotted mushroom of the Fair Folk, I call to you to awaken to yourself and to your many powers. You bring trance and vision. You bring the flight of the spirit and open the second sight. You, daughter of the underworld, are altogether good. Bright grand-mother, open the gates within me, that I might know the truth. Bring vision and inspiration to all who breathe you in. Bring the underworld up to me and carry my wishes down with your smoke.

Cherry, childhood tree-friend, I call you into living beauty. Your roots twist into the deepest Earth, and your branches stretch to touch the Heavens. You give fruit and flower, you nourish both body and soul. Ground me in your mighty roots, and lift me up to the heavens in a vessel of your beautiful blossom.

The Middle World

The Middle World is where our bodies live and where our consciousnesses are most of the time. Many, many types of spirits live here. We living crea-tures are by far the most common kind, but there are also many strong discorporate ambassador spirits from groups of living creatures, such as American Black Bear, Oak, or even Rosaceae, a wonderful, magical spirit of a large family of flowering plants that includes roses, apples, strawber-ries, hawthorn, and many other fairy-friendly plants. Additionally, there are many coteries and collectives of unembodied spirits, such as the Elemen-tals and Fairy Courts. The Middle World is also home to the genii locorum, the spirits of places both great and small. These local spirits are extremely powerful allies, and the spirits of your home are likely to want to support you, as long as you support them.

OFFERING INCENSE FOR MOTHER NATURE
& THE MIDDLE WORLD

Far more so than the other worlds, the Middle World is our home. Whether or not you, like me, are a dirty, tree-hugging Earth worshipper, there are many reasons you might want to make offerings to Mother Nature and the collective spirits of the Middle World. This incense was originally designed to accompany Orphic Hymn #10, for Physis, which is included below. However, it is excellent as an all-purpose offering for any avatar of Nature and the Middle World.

> 3 parts cedar, or another aromatic wood
>
> 1 part rose
>
> 1 part kitchen sage
>
> 1 part tobacco

Here are some more examples of awakening invocations you can use as inspiration to write your own:

> Cedar, tall and straight, you are the pillar that holds up the sky, and your great roots secure the foundations of the Earth. You are ever-green, everpure, and altogether good. Lend me your strength and shade me under your mighty boughs, benevolent protector.

> Rose, queen of flowers, beauty incarnate, you are the glory of creation and the ephemeral love that unites all things.

> Sage, green sage, you are the smell of home and hearth, the very essence of family and community. You make mouths water and minds wander. Open my senses to experience the goodness of creation and spread your cloak of protection and purity around me, defeating any miasma or pollution.

> Tobacco, sacred smoke, you awaken the spirit and bring life to the senses. You unite all living things in peace and community. Tobacco, sacred smoke, I give thanks for the wonder of the world.

Orphic Hymn to Physis

Incline to our prayer and grant us your favor,

Physis, All-Matter, divine Mother Nature.

Much-mechanical matrix of clockwork creation,

Ancient Great Mother, accept our libation!

Celestial Anassa, lustrous and endless,

Indomitable dictator, all-conquering empress,

Almighty mistress of the mountainous breast,

Nursing the world, happy and blest.

Imperishable Protogeneia, exulted of old,

Sung forth by the night stars, their numbers untold:

Silent galaxies whirl on light-leaping feet,

The pitter-patter of matter to time's tick-tock beat.

Pure cosmic mother, unbounded, eternal,

Font of all gods, heavenly and infernal.

Common to all, but uncommonly unique

All-pervading quintessence of all that we seek.

Full-blossoming weaver of natural tapestry,

Self-made and fatherless, poly-mythic majesty

Head of hegemony, life-bearing maiden

Victorious charm-weaver, seductive all-daimon.

Self-sufficient founder of multiverse reality:

Ethereal, material, and abyssal locality.

Bitter to the sinner, but sweet to the saint,

All-wise, all-generous, all-giving, all-great,

Queen for forever, rich ripening savior,

Growth-promoting immortal divine liberator.

Father and mother, nurturing all-fruitful womb,

Giving birth to the seasons, coaxing blossoms to bloom.

You crafted the cosmos and you wove the waves,

Your perpetual motion spins nights into days.

Everlastingly circling, quick-flowing, whirling,

Fluid-formed shape-changer, eternally swirling.

Mover and shaker of every eternity,

Worldly-wise essence, much-honored deity:

Enthroned, scepter-bearing, growling with power,

Mountains rumble your presence, roaring out fire.

All-dominating mistress of life without end,

Future-seeing foremother on whom all depend.

Truly, to everyone you are everything,

And from your immortal being all fates spring.

Good Goddess, Great Mother, we humbly request

You guide us through life, happy and blest.

Bring every good thing, each in its season,

Peace, health and prosperity, wisdom and reason.

ECOREGIONAL INCENSE

This is among the most difficult recipes in this book—and also the most flexible—because it will vary drastically based on the season and location you are making it in. The goal is to capture the essence of the natural world around you, so it's important that you use plants local to where you are. Making this incense begins with a walk and a collecting basket. Gather anything that smells good or catches your eye. If you're not sure what it is, take a picture of the whole plant and a close-up of the leaves to help you identify it once you get home. Keep a particular eye out for berries, artemisia, flowers, conifer needles, resins, and herbs, all of which should be harvestable in most ecoregions, including urban ones. If, for whatever reason, you can't collect all your own ingredients, here is a basic recipe you can make from things you can buy at a health store. Add your own local plants to it. Experiment to find what works best for you. Every time you make this incense, it will be a little different. The mixture below is a summer blend here in the Eastern Woodlands. With the exception of the honey, I grow everything on this list in my yard.

> 1 part native resin (I use pine.)
>
> 1 part pine or other needles
>
> 3 parts native artemisia (Here in the Eastern Woodlands, I use mugwort.)
>
> 1 part dried berries or other fruit (I use mulberries, elderberries, or crab apples, depending on the season.)
>
> 2 parts pleasant-smelling wild herbs and wildflowers (In my most recent batch, I used red and white clover, chamomile, and calendula.)
>
> 1 part spicebush berries
>
> Local honey to bind (It is particularly important to use local honey in this recipe. If you cannot get local honey, omit the honey entirely, and use extra fruit instead.)

Awaken each ingredient as you gather it. Here are some examples:

Pine, your smell is the smell of the forest; you are the King of Trees. No unclean thing can be in your presence, for you are altogether true and good. You grow tall and straight, connecting the Heavens and the

Underworld, but you, yourself, live with me, here at the center of the universe, the living heart of the Middle World. I burn you as an offering for all spirits of the Middle World. Make open the roads between us for knowledge and conversation. Pine, every spirit delights in your scent; become for them every delightful thing.

Artemisia, Queen of the Greenling Wood, I call on you to awaken to yourself. Herb of vision, herb of communion, open my mind to know, my eyes to see, and my ears to hear. Open my heart to work with the spirits. Una, eldest of spirits, I call on you to intercede with spirits for me. I burn you as an offering for the spirits of the Great Forest. Make easy the way for me to travel, and also for them. May you be for them every delicious thing. All who are beneficent may stay to visit. All who wish me ill must be satisfied with this offering and depart.

Elder Mother, Green of the Darkling Wood, look kindly on me. Your blossoms are the white stars that shine by night. Your berries are the fructified essence of healing. You bring beauty, healing, and protection to all who come to you with respect. You teach the craft of the witches, and the secrets of the deep wood. I burn you as an offering for spirits of the Nighttime Forest. Make easy the way for us to communicate. We offer them healing and blessing, and accept such in return from those who would offer it.

Flowers of the meadow, the bee's delight, blossoms and nectar and the sweet essence of the honey, you are the beauty of the Land, bright jewels of life and light and love. I burn you as an offering for all the spirits of the Middle World, that you bring them delight as you have brought it to me. Form garlands of smoke to crown them, and be the sweetness that delights their tongues. May you be transformed into every wonderful thing.

THE SPIRITS OF THE SEASONS & THE SEASONAL COURTS

Some types of spirits like the genii locorum are rooted in space and exercise meaningful power only in certain places. Other types of spirits are rooted in time. Of these, perhaps the most famous are the seasonal courts among the Good Neighbors. Although some recognize only two courts, the Seelie and Unseelie, for the most part, I work with four seasonal courts. As with almost all spirit classifications, the courts are not strict categories; many spirits flit around the edges of several courts but belong to none, and others change shape to infiltrate them all. The seasonal courts are not ruled over by astrological phenomena; they live and die with the weather. The dates of their coming and going cannot always be predicted, but they can easily be observed. As spirits of the Middle World, and ones intimately connected with the rhythm of seasons, the courts can be very, very different in different locations. What follows is not a teaching on traditional British/ Celtic fairy lore, but a teaching on the seasons and their spirits.

Spring

As the soil warms, the rains return, and the trees begin to flower, the Spring Court takes power. Spirits of spring tend to be curious and playful, but a little shy. They are great lovers of all things beautiful and are easily swayed by offerings of original poetry, songs, and theater. Perform for them what you created over the long winter inside. They are lavish in their blessings for those whom they favor, but can be cruel to those who displease them. They generally delight in young children, but can be prone to teaching rude or selfish older children manners, sometimes in unpleasant—but rarely dangerous—ways. Plant fruiting trees, crocuses, or other early-blooming pollinator favorites to make a good impression. Where I live in Pennsylvania, the spirits of the Spring Court begin to poke their heads out in early April and are usually in the full glory of their reign by May Day. By the summer solstice, the Spring Court is receding, giving way to their hot-blooded summer cousins.

This incense is an excellent offering for all spirits of the Spring Court, but most especially for their blossom-bedecked May Queen. She is known by many names: Una, Maia, Flora, She of the Wildflower Meadow, and a hundred, hundred other names. This incense is great for any work related to abundance, prosperity, fertility, fecundity, marriage, family, gardens, or a happy and healthy sex life. However, it's also great as a mood setter; it is a delightful and refreshing way to bring in the spring, especially when you've been cooped up. Open the windows to let the bad air out and burn this incense to chase it on its way. The proportions can vary tremendously depending on the exact plants, where you source your materials, how fresh they are, and your own personal taste.

3 parts frankincense or other resin for the warmth of the sun

3 parts rose for love, beauty, and floral splendor

2 parts damiana as a tonic to get those spring juices flowing

1 part clover leaves for the fecundity of the Land and the growing green

1 part dried hawthorn berries from last summer's harvest

1 part apple or other fruit blossoms for the favor of the Fair Folk and for a rich and luscious harvest (As you pick the blossoms, keep in mind how doing so helps the tree build stronger roots. How does this apply in your own life?)

Honey to bind (This recipe particularly benefits from local honey.)

I use this slightly modified traditional hymn to bless this incense, which is best made on May Day:

Bring flowers of the rarest,

Bring blossoms the fairest,

From garden and woodland and hillside and dale;

Our full hearts are swelling,

Our glad voices telling

The praise of the loveliest flower of the vale.

O Lady, we crown thee with blossoms today,

Queen of Fairies and Queen of the May!

O Lady, we crown thee with blossoms today,

Queen of Fairies and Queen of the May!

Depending on the flavor of May Queen you want, you might substitute "Queen of Heaven" or "Queen of the Spring" for "Queen of Fairies." The traditional line is "Queen of Angels." Where I have "Lady," the traditional hymn sings to "Mary."

Summer

The Summer Court is the most beneficent and human-loving of the courts, although even they can be vicious when provoked. In my experience, the Summer Court is the most traditional, formal, and hierarchical; be sure to be very proper and respectful. They are, in my experience, especially fond of baked goods and physical offerings, like picking up litter or planting trees. At this time of year, there is much labor to be done. The Summer Court delights in music and dancing even more than the Spring Court. They also love a good wrestling match or sword fight.

The Summer Queen—who, of course, is really just *the Queen* in a different costume—rejoices in many names: Titania, the Foxglove Queen, the Berry Queen, Lady of Elphame, She of the Green. She is bedecked in flowers of all colors and lusciously dripping fruits. In my vision, she sometimes wears a catskin, the traditional costume of the Maenads, and travels with a pack of mountain lions. This incense may be used as an offering to the Summer Queen and all spirits of summer. It is a nice accompaniment to spells for prosperity, although unless you are a farmer, it would not be my go-to spell for that. I sometimes burn it during parties; it is happy and refreshing.

> 3 parts pine resin
>
> 2 parts citrus peel (I like clementine for this.)
>
> 1 part dried berries (I usually use mulberries.)
>
> 1 part vervain
>
> 1 part mint

Autumn

As the apples ripen and the grass begins to yellow, the Autumn Court makes their appearance, led by the beautiful Apple Queen. Autumnal spirits tend to be wise, protective, and beneficent, but can be fiercely malicious when provoked to anger. Many of them are excellent teachers of sorcery and make powerful allies and sagacious counselors when won over to a cause. These spirits appreciate hard work and deep silence. Bring in the harvest, put the gardens to bed, and sit quietly among the fallen leaves, listening to the rattling wind. To win their favor, carpet your garden with all the fallen leaves you can lay hold of, creating a rich, deep blanket for the cooling soil. Get to know the teeming chthonic biome. Here in the Eastern Woodlands, the Autumn Court's ascent often ends abruptly with the first snowfall. Traditionally, this was often near Halloween, but it's been moving later and later year by year.

2 parts resin for the precious warmth of the receding sun

2 parts dried apples for the bounty of the harvest (If you grow other autumn fruits, like pears, substitute them.)

1 part aromatic wood (Something local is nice.)

1 part cinnamon for warmth and coziness

1 part cloves for autumnal color

1 part spicebush or allspice for that "pumpkin pie" smell

1 part tobacco for an earthy bonfire smell

This incense makes me think of all the things I love about autumn: falling leaves, thick sweaters, chai lattes, leather coats, demon lovers, and necromancy. It's primarily intended as an offering for spirits of the Autumn Court, including the Apple Queen, and most red birds.

Winter

While I originally designed it for New Year's Eve, this incense is excellent for the winter solstice and all her associated holidays. It is also good whenever you want to mark the end of one cycle and the beginning of another. It can be used as an offering to the spirits of the Winter Court and is also well-favored by most house spirits. It is particularly nice as an offering to Granny Winter, an ambassador spirit from the same coterie as the Norse goddess Hel, the Germanic Perchta, the fairy-tale Frau Holle, the Elderberry Mother, Mother Goose, and many others. This incense is very happy and pleasant-smelling and can help set a nice vibe for holiday parties and other get-togethers.

3 parts frankincense

2 parts cedar

1 part rosemary

1 part cinnamon

1 part citrus peel

1 part elderberries

The frankincense is used in this recipe primarily for its solar aspects. It brings light to dark days, while uplifting and inspiring courage. If you're making this as a Christmas incense, you might want to awaken its connection with the three Wise Men, and thus with the infant Christ. If for Chanukah, consider awakening it to ever increase the light of the world.

The cedar in this recipe helps to build bridges over the chasms of death. I mean this in two ways: (1) it opens a way for the ancestors to join you, and (2) it smooths a path to let go of things that are holding you back. Ask Grandmother Cedar to open your senses so that you can perceive new possibilities.

Rosemary is here to clarify the vision and also for its delicious smell, triggering memories of holiday feasts both personal and mythic. The cinnamon warms the mixture, adding the comfort of a cozy fire, with a hint of spice to keep things moving forward. The citrus peel helps to cut through illusions and adds a younger and more immediate note to the more eternal solar energy we found in the frankincense. Finally, the elderberries are here to impart some robustness against winter illnesses and lighten the heart against winter blues. More importantly, they are used for their connection to Granny Winter and her house of healing.

OFFERING INCENSES FOR ELEMENTALS

There are, the ancients teach, five elements necessary for life to thrive: the life-giving soul of the Aether, the life-giving breath of Air, the life-giving refreshment of Water, the life-giving warmth of Fire, and the life-giving nourishment of the Earth. The spirits of these elements are among humans' oldest incorporeal allies. Remember that these are discorporate elemental spirits. For example, "Earth" below does not mean Terra, nor does it mean soil. It is a nonphysical spirit associated with the Platonic elemental, Earth.

Elemental Earth is the densest element. Like solid matter, it can be seen, tasted, smelled, felt, and heard. It is cold and dry. Earth is the body and other material things. Anthropomorphic ambassador spirits of the Earth include the gnomes, pygmies, dwarves, dryads, and many types of Good Neighbors. These spirits are often patient and reliable, but sometimes inflexible or close-minded. Earth's weapon is the shield, and its vessel is the spade. Earth's symbolic animal is most often the bull, but sometimes the elephant or turtle.

 Elemental Water is less dense than elemental Earth. Like liquid water, it can be seen, felt, and heard, but it has no smell or taste. It is cold and wet. Water is associated with the heart, the blood, the emotions, and all chemical processes within the body. Anthropomorphic ambassador spirits of the Waters include the undines, nereids, mermaids, and many types of sea people. These spirits are often compassionate and wise, but they can also be irrational and vicious. Water's weapon is the chalice, and her vessel is the cauldron. Water's symbolic animal is most often the fish, but sometimes the human or mermaid.

 Elemental Fire can be seen, heard, smelled and felt but it has no taste. It is hot and dry. Fire is associated with the spirit and the passions. Anthropomorphic ambassador spirits of the Flames include djinn, salamanders, vulcans, and many other types of Fire beings. Fire spirits are usually brave and exciting, but they can also be belligerent and short-tempered. Fire's weapon is the staff, and its vessel is the torch. Fire's symbolic animal is usually the lion, but sometimes a dragon.

Elemental Air can be felt and heard, but not perceived with the other senses. It is warm and dry. Air is associated with the mind, and all the activities thereof, including communication, invention, and academics. Anthropomorphic ambassador spirits of the Air include the sylphs, sylvestris, satyrs, and many other types of Fair Folk. Air spirits are most often smart and quick, although they can also be flaky or condescending. Air's weapon is the sword, and its vessel is the drum. Most often, the symbolic animal of Air is the eagle, but sometimes other birds are used.

 Elemental Aether, also called Quintessence or Void, can be heard, but sensed in no other way. Anthropomorphic ambassador spirits of the Aether include angels, aliens, demons, and many types of Outsiders. These types of spirits are more often found in the Upper and Lower Worlds than here in the Middle. Aetheric spirits tend to be powerful, inscrutable, and remote. They are often incomprehensible, disquieting, and deeply, deeply weird.

An Offering Incense for All Elemental Beings

This incense is designed as an offering to all elemental beings. In order to involve all of the senses, I've included ingredients that hiss and pop and others that tend to spark. Be careful to burn this incense on a large ceramic plate or other fireproof surface. For this recipe, it's best to add the ingredients to the charcoal one at a time, rather than premixing them.

For Fire, frankincense, the light and warmth of the sun made solid (If you grind some of it very fine, it will spark and flame when you add it to the charcoal.)

For Water, coarsest sea salt—the conductivity and fluidity of the sea made solid (You can also drop the tiniest splash of water on for a hiss

and some steam, but be careful not to put the charcoal out. The salt
will pop.)

For Air, rose—the ideal ephemerality of the wind made solid (Use whole
rose petals, and they'll lift a little while they burn.)

For Earth, cedar—the reliable stability of the land beneath our feet (Clap
or stomp three times.)

Elemental Earth & Earth Elementals

Earth is, as Hesiod would have it, the "wide-bosomed foundation of all."
When thought of magically, the realm of Earth includes our physical health,
our physical home, wealth, and family stability. The most common type of
Earth magic I do is long-term wealth building, but it's also excellent for
grounding, home protection, and some kinds of healing. The Earth elementals I work with most often are the dwarves. There is no denying that these
Earth elementals are our close kin; they are the most anthropomorphic of
elementals. This incense was originally created for Norðri, Suðri, Austri,
and Vestri, four arch-dwarves who hold up the pillars of the Earth, but it
is equally good for all dwarves, all Earth elementals, or as an offering to
Earth itself. I like to burn this on a pile of native soil.

3 parts mugwort or other artemisia as a base to open the senses and
encourage spirit manifestation

2 parts juniper or other conifer needles for their connection with the
forest and as a sacred World Tree

1 part thyme for courage and strength

1 part dried button or other mushrooms to lend a deep and slightly dirt-
like scent

1 part crab apples or other dried fruit for the bounty of the Land

Elemental Air & Air Elementals

More than any other element, Air connects us to every other living thing
on Earth. Breathe in, knowing that the air you are breathing was exhaled
by the trees. Breath out, and your exhalations give plants life. We are all
of us united in an eternal cycle of respiration. Air is ephemeral, but all-
encompassing and ever-permeating. If ever you doubt your devotion to

the spirits of the winds, hold your breath until you remember it again. Air magic is excellent for all types of academic magic, as well as many types of career magic. Use it on your résumé and before you make a big presentation. Personally, however, I most often work with the sylphs as allies in political and environmental malefica. I live within sight of the last remaining Carnegie Steel mill, and my neighborhood has some of the worst air quality in the country. For this reason, I rarely burn incense for the spirits of the Air; it is unwise to work for clean air over a smokestack. More often, I use this blend as a potpourri or an oil, but you can also burn it.

> 4 parts peppermint for clarity
>
> 2 parts bay leaf for brightness
>
> 2 parts citrus peel for crispness
>
> 1 part star anise for the piercing fierceness of the winds

Elemental Water & Water Elementals

Water is the wiliest and slipperiest of elements, flooding and flowing into every shape. It is the universal solvent; it dissolves obstacles and treasures alike. When thought of esoterically, water magic is most often about managing emotions and social dynamics. I most frequently use it for healing psychic trauma, but it is also excellent for lubricating any kind of social interaction with another person from a job interview to a marriage. The water elementals I work with most often are the nereids, a type of sea nymph or mermaid in the court of Poseidon. In particular, I work with Amphitrite, the goddess of salt and lover of Poseidon. In my experience, the water elementals are the most diverse and populous of the elemental tribes. This incense is also excellent as a bath. Put the mixture in a cloth bag, tightly tied closed. Add generous salt to the bath.

> 2 parts hyssop for the cleansing power of the sea
>
> 1 part lemon for the clarity of clean rain
>
> 1 part rose for the beauty of love and emotional clarity
>
> 1 part damiana for emotional healing and love
>
> Honey to bind

Elemental Fire & Fire Elements

Fire is often the most difficult of the elements to control and the most mysterious. Fire sparks almost instantly into existence and fizzles out just as fast. It is, in many ways, the least material of the elements, but also the most alive. Magically, Fire is often related to will, passion, art, and sex. It is a good choice when you need protection, power, or motivation. This incense is very similar to a traditional recipe called Fiery Wall of Protection and can be used for that purpose with the spell here.

> 4 parts dragon's blood resin for its fiery red color and association with dragons
>
> 3 parts cinnamon for the comforting warmth of the family hearth
>
> 2 parts tarragon to open the senses, encourage spirit manifestation, and for its association with dragons
>
> 1 part whole black peppercorns for heat
>
> Honey to bind

FIERY WALL OF PROTECTION SPELL

This spell provides powerful protection against malefic influence, but tends to be rather short-lived. It should be cast in response to a specific situation and not as an all-purpose prophylactic. For other protection options, see the chapter on spellwork.

YOU WILL NEED

> A recent photo of the enemy you desire protection from
>
> Hair, blood, worn clothing, or other personal concerns from the target (DNA samples are best.) (Optional)
>
> A prepared censer, with charcoal, and a way to light it
>
> About half a cup of the Fire elemental incense or a similar blend
>
> A paper grocery bag cut open and laid flat, writing-side down, *or* another large piece of paper
>
> A white candle (A tea light is fine.)
>
> Charcoal from a large fire *or* a large black magic marker

WHAT TO DO

◆ Center yourself, and enter into magical space, time, and consciousness.

◆ Attach the personal concerns to the photo, and baptize it with the name of your enemy.

◆ Put the candle and the censer in the center of the paper. Light the charcoal, but do not yet add incense or light the candle.

◆ Using the charcoal or the marker, draw three concentric circles around the candle.

◆ Make a circular wall of extra incense on top of the middle circle.

◆ Place the photo on the far side of the circle, so you have to look over the candle to see it.

◆ Prepare to enchant.

◆ Light the candle, and drop the first pinch of incense onto the charcoal.

◆ Say something like:

Scorching Fire, Warlike son of Heaven,

Fiercest of thy brethren,

Who, like Moon and Sun, decides lawsuits—

Judge my case, hand down the verdict!

Erect a wall of flames between me and NAME, who has bewitched me;

Burn, O Fire, NAME should they seek to do me ill;

Burn them, O Fire!

Scorch them, O Fire!

Take hold of them, O Fire!

Consume them, O Fire!

Destroy them, O Fire!*

---

* This incantation is strongly modeled on Thorkild Jacobsen's translation of Murqual Tablet IV.

♦ While speaking, fan the smoke around to make a vortex, feeling the wall of flames grow up to surround you in protection. At the end of the incantation, push the smoke, using hands and breath, toward the target as hard as possible. Imaging you are a dragon, breathing fire. Let the candle burn down, and then gather up the incense wall and the ashes of burnt incense. Ideally, sprinkle them across the threshold of your home, and carry a pinch in your left pocket.

HOUSE SPIRITS

In every era, in every culture, the wise have known that we share our spaces and our lives with all manner of spirits. Among the most important of these spirits—although frequently overlooked—are the spirits we share our homes with. In ancient days these were often called the family gods. Following ancient custom, in this book I will consistently use the word *family* to refer to all occupants of a home, no matter whether they are officially related. Family gods cover a wide range of spirits, including deified heroes, saints, and other Mighty Dead, guardian spirits, and the land spirits of the local area. These family gods can be kept on the dining table, either in the form of statues or in a decorative ceramic jar, and fed tiny pinches of family meals. In addition to these intentional offerings, any food that falls to the floor is, by custom, theirs. In Latin, these spirits are called Lares or Penates, in Anglo-Saxon they are Cofgodas, and in Hebrew they are called תרפים (teraphim).

A modern type of spirit housemates are those my family calls hobs, but which are known by countless other names as well. Almost all scholars agree that these creatures are the family gods and ancestors gone under cover to survive Christianity. Hobs are spirits; they do not have a fixed physical form, but they most often appear as small men, wizened with age, often wearing green or red. They sometimes also appear as old women or small children.

It should be obvious why it's good to build a strong and friendly relationship with your house spirits; you literally live with them. A house with happy hobs stays cleaner, decays more slowly, and is peaceful and healthier to live in. Clean, well-maintained, peaceful, healthy homes keep hobs happy. Regular offerings are one great way to forge a strong relationship with your hobs. This incense will not only serve as an offering to strengthen your hobs, but also promote a peaceful, happy, and cozy home.

> 1 part local resin to drive away all evil influences (If possible, collect this near your home.)
>
> 1 part local aromatic wood to bring the peace of the forest into your home
>
> 1 part cinnamon to keep your home warm, safe, and delicious
>
> 1 part lemon peel to drive away all evil influences
>
> 1 part clover for luck, health, and wealth

A complementary floor wash may be made by adding cinnamon essential oil to lemon Pine-Sol.

The Underworld

The Underworld is home to a wide variety of types of spirits for whom you may want to make incense offerings, including the chthonic gods and the dead, who are generally grouped into two categories: the Mighty Dead, who are adored and venerated by many, many people, and the Beloved Dead, such as your own ancestors, with whom you have a more personal connection.

OFFERING INCENSE FOR THE QUEEN(S) OF HELL & ALL UNDERWORLD SPIRITS

This incense was specifically designed for Persephone of Eleusis, but it is equally appropriate for almost any goddess who rules over the dead, including Helle, Proserpina, Ereshkigal, Maman Brigitte, Santa Muerte, Our Lady of Sorrows, and many, many others. While many people are scared of these goddesses, I find them essentially and eternally compassionate, welcoming, and healing. These goddesses are always in some sense dual. They are the goddess of death, but also of rebirth. Particularly in temperate climates, they are often associated with the cycle of the seasons.

> 3 parts mugwort to open the psychic senses and thin the veil for spirit communication

2 parts myrrh or another resin as a rich and special offering (Myrrh is
    particularly suitable because of its funereal associations.)
1 part poppy seeds for their association with sleep, trance, and
    underworld travel (They're also especially sacred to Persephone.)
1 part orris root appropriate to the underworld's eternal peace for its
    delicately floral and long-lasting fixative scent (Like all roots, it grows
    underground.)

PSYCHOPOMPS

Psychopomps are gods who help guide the spirits of the recently dead.
There are many to choose from. They should have the following mythological qualities:

They traditionally appear on grave markers and in funeral rites.

They guide the dead.

They know the name of every spirit.

They can walk in all three worlds.

Most, but not all, psychopomps, also have the following characteristics:

They carry a torch.

They are tricksters.

They are shape-shifters.

They have wings.

They are accompanied by or shape-shift into domesticated animals.

They are accompanied by or shape-shift into a large flying bird or a
    large flock of smaller birds, usually black or nocturnal.

I most often work with Hermes Chthonios, an underworld face of the
Greek god of crossroads, travel, translation, games, cleverness, thievery,
and every kind of intersectionality. Just a few examples of other excellent
choices to fill this role are Hekate (the Greek goddess of liminality), White
Stag, Anubis (an Egyptian death god), Yew Tree, Jesus (with whom you
are probably familiar), and American Bison. If, in life, you only ever work

with one psychopomp, it is likely that they will help to guide you when it is your turn to walk the Long Road.

> 2 parts pine or another resin for the light, heat, and pop of the torch
>
> 1 part mint, strewn on the road beneath your feet
>
> 1 part tobacco for sacred smoke along the Long Road
>
> 1 part mugwort to open the ways and ease any pain
>
> Honey to bind

OFFERING INCENSE FOR THE MIGHTY DEAD

Who Are the Mighty Dead?

The Mighty Dead are simply those dead humans who retain a high level of personal coherence long after their death. Heroes, saints, and revered tribal ancestors are all types of the Mighty Dead. These are the dead who are most able to operate in our world. As I understand it, a dead person's ability to interact with the living world is partly a matter of skill and partly a matter of linkage. People who could talk to the dead when they were alive are often those who can most easily talk to the living once they are dead. More powerfully determinative, however, is their linkage to the world of the living. Ancestors and others among the Beloved Dead have links to the world only in those who love them. They can have great power in the lives of their descendants both literal or metaphoric, but have quite limited impact outside of that. Those spirits who have links to a large number of humans are more able to act in the world at large. These are the Mighty Dead.

At the most basic, what we have to offer to the dead is our interaction with them, which gives them a foothold toward becoming mighty. What they have to offer us varies based on who they are. Everyone among the Mighty Dead has enough to offer that many, many people have kept their names known and their stories told for a very long time. That's nearly always worth investigating. Not every two people will get along, and that's just as true when one of them is dead as it is among the living. Not all among the Mighty Dead will appeal to you, and among those who do, there's no guarantee that all of them will want to work with you. I think about it like dating: sometimes they're just not that into you.

Incense for the Mighty Dead

> 4 parts frankincense or another resin for a bright and sacred base
>
> 2 parts cedar or another aromatic wood to act as a World Tree, but also for its particular association with the dead
>
> 1 part rose for beauty and love and to lend an elegant air to the incense
>
> 1 part cloves for wealth and power and to lend a regal air to the incense
>
> Honey to bind as well as to provide a thick, luxurious quality to the smoke and to sweeten it, making this an enticing offering for the dead

A Ritual for Honoring the Mighty Dead

This is not the only way to honor the Mighty Dead; every culture and every practitioner will have their own methods. You'll develop your own way, which works for you, with practice. This is just one example to get you started.

YOU WILL NEED

> About 2 square feet of table space
>
> A white tablecloth
>
> A head covering such as a scarf or veil that can be draped to restrict your field of vision
>
> A white candle
>
> Incense and a way to burn it
>
> A glass of water
>
> About an hour
>
> An ikon or other picture of the Mighty Dead you wish to honor (You can do a whole bunch at once, but it's better if they each have their own image.)

WHAT TO DO

♦ Clean your table, lay out the cloth, and arrange the other items on it in a pleasing fashion.

- Position yourself and your head covering to restrict your field of vision to the altar.

- Enter into magical space, time, and consciousness by any method.

- Light the candle and the incense.

- Greet the Mighty Dead. Call them by flowery titles and describe what you love best about them. This is exactly the same as awakening ingredients, but even easier, because the thing you're awakening is a human-person, with a name and a story, which is much easier to understand than a plant-person, because you are also a human-person with a name and a story.

- Explain that you are offering them light, heat, and flame. Explain that you are offering cool, clean water. Explain that you are offering the smoke, the scent, and the incense itself.

- Tell them why you have come (To commune with them as friends and allies? To ask a favor? To do your religious duty? Why are you doing this ritual?).

- Quiet your mind, and do your very best to watch, listen, sense, and feel for a response. If the incense runs out, light more. Breathe it in. Blow it onto the ikons. Allow its swirling to transmit visions to you. Do this for about forty-five minutes, or until you are too overwhelmed to continue.

- When you are done, thank the spirits who communicated with you, and give your good wishes to all the spirits.

- Return to regular space, time, and consciousness.

- Take notes on your experiences. Like dreams, ritual experiences can fade fast.

OFFERINGS FOR THE ANCESTORS

Trigger Warning

There is no way to talk about ancestors without dealing with many difficult subjects. I've tried my very best to be sensitive but still straightforward about the many, many ways our relationships with our ancestors are fraught and complicated. These include both cultural issues like race, ethnicity, colonization, and enslavement and more personal issues like incest and abuse. Everyone's roots grow in dirt.

There Is Only One Family Tree on Earth

Before we talk about working with ancestors of blood, I want to speak first about a simple but profound truth: All living things on Earth are kin. It's not entirely clear how many times life came to be on our planet, but all currently living organisms share common ancestry. Modern science suggests that the Last Universal Common Ancestor (LUCA) of modern Earth life lived sometime between four and four and a half billion years ago. Life is nearly as old as Earth herself. We don't know much about LUCA; xe appears to have been an asexual single-cell life-form similar to, but simpler than, modern bacteria. Most likely, LUCA lived in the boiling hot deep-sea vents of the primordial sea. In these liminal spaces the primordial fires of Earth's inner heart push molten rock up to meet the chilly ocean waters in spouts of life-giving air. It is a mistake to understand LUCA to be the first living creature on Earth. Xe almost certainly had company, but only xir descendants survived into the present day, becoming the vast, rich, beautiful, and multi-mysterious panoply of life we know today.

An Offering for the Ancestors & Beloved Dead

> 6 parts myrrh to provide a rich, warm, funereal base to this incense
>
> 2 parts cedar to function primarily as a World Tree in this recipe, in addition to cedar's resonance as a traditional offering to the dead
>
> 2 parts tobacco as another traditional offering for the dead
>
> 1 part cinnamon for a smell of home and family, as well as warmth, which the dead crave (Use slightly more if using cassia.)
>
> Honey to bind

This is the last recipe for which I'll be providing explicit awakening formulas. Remember, these are examples. You should be writing your own.

Myrrh, antidote, severe one of the flames,

Intercessor, reconciler, you who sets spirits ablaze.

Myrrh is your name among the profane

but I call to you now by your secret names:

I call Sarcophagus, Flesh-eater, the Scorcher of Hearts.

I call on you now, and charge you to depart,

Not to distant Araby, nor far Babylon,

But only to work my will as liaison:

Thrice-blest resin that hallows the dead,

Grief-releaser, who defends from leaden dread,

You are Helios's golden tears, shining sun shed:

Pour out the warmth of the heavens into the Land of the Dead.

Grandmother Cedar, mother of love and mother of might

Your branches reach up, up, up to the heights.

Your eternal trunks grow tall and proud,

your roots reach down, down, down under the ground.

You are the love of the living for the dead,

You calm the mind and clear the head,

You are altogether good and incorruptibly pure.

Please nourish my ancestors so they may endure.

Tobacco: clever, kind and altogether calm,

Your sweet smoke is life's good balm.

You ease the pains of each hard day,

And carry up the wishes of those who pray.

You ease sorrow and soothe anxiety,

Please feed the Ancestors in love and piety.

Cinnamon, cinnamon, spice of riches and joy

Awaken now and go as my envoy:

Cinnamon, cinnamon, burn sweet with heat,

And warm the souls of all you meet.

I call to you, Honey, remember your powers

You are the essence of nature gathered from flowers

The Knight of the Meadow, the rush-buzzing bee

Gathered you together and brought you to me.

Honey, sweet honey, you serve as the glue

That binds generations together: sure, pure, and true.

Setting Up an Ancestor Altar

Now that you've made an incense to offer them, I recommend setting up a place to burn it. An ancestor altar is a way to give your ancestors a physical purchase from which they can more easily interact with you and your life. There are many, many styles of ancestor altars. If any of the cultures of your recent ancestry have their own style, those are a good place to start researching. However, at a basic level, all of them work in the same ways. You will develop your own practice over time.

The first step in setting up an ancestor altar is choosing where to put it. A shelf or small table is fine, or the top of a bookcase or dresser. In my previous homes, mine was in an inherited cabinet. In the Witch House, we have a large ancestor altar in the basement, which is part of a larger altar for working with the dead and the gods of the dead. Ancestor altars can be super stealthy and are appropriate even in places where you don't want to make your witchy tendencies known; there is nothing suspicious about displaying photos and mementos of those we've loved and lost.

Whatever piece of furniture you choose, clean it thoroughly, both physically and magically. Wipe it down with a nice-smelling perfume or oil. Florida Water—a citrusy, floral, spicy cologne used a lot in both Hoodoo and Vudoun—is traditional, but I use Jean Naté—a citrusy, floral, spicy cologne my late mother wore. Once it's clean, lay a white cloth on top (optional, but traditional). If you have an inherited lace tablecloth, that is perfect. If your altar has an inside, you may want to paint it red, white, black, or any color that feels appropriate to you. You should also have a glass of clean water, which you should change out frequently—once a week is good, more if it's going dry or getting dirty. Most people say this should be in a white or clear glass, but I use a cobalt blue one I inherited from my mother. You'll probably also want a source of perpetual light, like an electric candle. What else goes on your ancestor altar varies dramatically from person to person, culture to culture, and tradition to tradition, but here are some broad suggestions.

DO INCLUDE

> **Photos** or other pictures of the departed
>
> **Incense** and a way to burn it
>
> **Religious paraphernalia** like ikons, idols, Bibles, etc.
>
> Food/drink **offerings**
>
> An **empty picture frame** or generic statue to represent unknown ancestors
>
> Small **stone skulls** and other memento mori
>
> **Dirt** or **pebbles** from graves or cremated **ashes**
>
> **Personal mementos** from recent ancestors, like jewelry and such (Pocket watches seem very popular. I am especially fond of eyeglasses, which

I use to see from their point of view. If your altar has drawers, they
are good places to keep this sort of thing, as well as photos and
documents. If not, consider getting some pretty boxes.)

Flowers, fake, fresh, or dried

Your own **death-preparation** documents such as medical directives, wills,
final testaments, and burial plans

DO NOT INCLUDE:

Salt (Small amounts, such as in food offerings, are okay.)

Iron (Small pieces, such as in jewelry, are okay.)

Photos of living people (Although the prohibitions on salt and iron are
common worldwide, they are nowhere near as universal as this
prohibition. Putting a photo of a living person on an ancestor altar will
draw them into the Land of the Dead in an unhealthy way.)

The Upper Worlds

GENERAL OFFERING INCENSE FOR THE HEAVENS

This incense is ideal for work with angels, planetary spirits, or other spirits
of the Heavens, especially if you are working with several of them at once.
It is particularly good for angels.

4 parts mixed resins

2 parts rose or another sweet flower

1 part cedar or another aromatic wood

Honey to bind

Individually awaken each ingredient by calling on its special properties
that you wish to incorporate. Grind the dry ingredients to a rough
powder, and mix together with sufficient honey to bind. Allow the
mixture to dry before packaging in a labeled, airtight container.

THE ARCHANGELS

The English word *angel* derives from the Greek word ἄγγελος (*angelos*). The Hebrew word for an angel is מלאך (*malakh*). All three words mean something like "who is sent"; in practice, they can mean ambassadors, translators, traders, intercessors, and other sorts of go-betweens, both human and otherwise. A less literal, but perhaps more instructive way to translate them is "functionary" or "bureaucrat." The angels I work with most often are the archangels of the four Earthly directions: Michael in the front, Gabriel in the back, Auriel on the right, and Raphael to the left. I work with these spirits both individually and as a collective, as in the protection spell below.

Archangels' Sacred Space

This spell is inspired by the traditional Jewish bedtime prayer, below, which is frequently sung as a lullaby.

B'shem Hashem	בְּשֵׁם הֲשֵׁם	In the name of the Name
Elohei Yisrael:	אֱלֹהֵי יִשְׂרָאֵל	The god of Israel:
mimini Michael	לְאָכִים יְנִימִין	Ahead is Michael
umismoli Gavriel,	לְאֵירְבַּג יְלֹאמְ'שִׁמוּ	Behind is Gabriel
umilfanai Auriel	לְאִירוּא יַנַפְלְמוּ	To the right Auriel
umeachorai Rafael,	לְאָפָר יַרוֹחָאֵמוּ	To the left Raphael
v'al roshi	יְשֹׁאר לַעְו	And above my head
Shechinat El	שׁ כִּנִַת א-ל.	the Divine Presence.

In the spell, we'll be using this same configuration of angels to construct a container for sacred space; that is to say, to cast a circle. Begin by preparing yourself and your space; you should both be clean and orderly. Arrange four censers in a circle. In the east, prepare frankincense for Michael (God-like) and in the west, cedar for Gabriel (Mighty). In the south, prepare cinnamon for Auriel (Light), and in the north, rosemary for Raphael (Healer). Stand in the center and prepare yourself. Recite or sing the prayer above in Hebrew or English, lighting the incense as you go. Sit in the middle, and experience the smells coming together. Spin, dance, move through the space, seeing how the fragrance is different in different places, experiencing the angels both individually and collectively. You and your body are the mechanism by which these energies are mixed; be sure all four smokes reach every corner of the room. If you own a feather fan, this is the time to use it! You can use this sacred space for other ritual work or to meditate or simple be in. When the censers have burned out and the smoke has settled, walk the perimeter of the room counterclockwise, sealing it. If you wish, while you walk you can say something like: "By the power of the two by two: Fourfold Forces, make it true!"

Archangels' Offering Incense

When you want to make an offering to the archangels without going through the whole ritual, you can use this incense blend. I recommend charging this incense in the center of the sacred space described above, but that is not required. The ratios of ingredients below are entirely about how fast the different ingredients burn.

> 3 parts frankincense for Michael, who carries the flaming sword
>   of truth
>
> 2 parts cedar for Gabriel, who carries the trumpet of revelation
>
> 1 part cinnamon chips for Auriel, who carries the torch of illumination
>
> 1 part rosemary for Raphael, who carries the chalice of healing

The Planets

The seven classical planets are among the most popular and traditional of magical allies. In European and Middle Eastern cultures, their virtues are relatively consistent cross-culturally, but their nature is not as universal as you might expect. Our Western understanding of the planets appears to have its roots in the ancient Near East, although since that is where literacy developed, it is difficult to establish their history before that. The seven luminous bodies we'll discuss in this chapter, usually referred to as the classical planets, are those objects that move through the night sky visible to the unaided eye from the surface of the Earth.

An Introduction to the Seven Classical Planets

☽ The Moon is the planet of the night, the subconscious, intuition, female lust, travel, and changeability. By extension, it is understood to be in alignment with femininity, luxury, dreams, all types of trance work, and most types of magic. Its colors are purple, gray, and silver. Its metal is silver, and its day is appropriately named Monday.

☿ Mercury is the planet of the intellect, swiftness, athletics, and both theft and commerce. By extension, it is also associated with the information age, trickery, merchants (which are named for Mercury), and literacy/education. Mercury's color is orange, and its traditional metal is quicksilver, although how you're supposed to carve a pentacle in liquid mercury I've never understood. These days, many magicians associate it with aluminum. Mercury's day is Wednesday, which derives its English name from the Germanic Wodan. Its symbol is the caduceus wand.

♀ Venus is the planet of procreation, beauty, love, friendship, green growing things, and luxury. By extension, it is also associated with all fertility, emotion, glamour, social skills, and status. Its color is emerald green and its metal copper, which was mined on the island of Cyprus sacred to the goddess Venus. Its day is Friday, which in English is named for the Norse goddess Freya. Venus's symbol is the mirror.

☉ The Sun is the power of radiance, healing, vision, and the source of life-sustaining energy. By extension, it is also associated with the ego, charisma, peace, and youth. Its color is yellow or gold, its metal gold, and its day, logically, is Sunday.

♂ Mars is the planet of war, conflict, justice (not mercy), and lust. By extension, it is also associated with victory, competition, impregnation, and other acts of strength. Its color is red, its metal iron, and its day Tuesday, which has its English name from Tyr, a Norse warrior god. Its symbol is the spear.

♃ Jupiter is in many ways the opposite of Saturn. Whereas Saturn is most often worked with to direct power inward, Jupiter is all about expansion. This is the planet of growth, kingship, grace (divine gifts), health, and material success. By extension, it is often associated with money, business, and command. Its color is blue, and its metal is tin. Jupiter's day is Thursday, which, in English, is named after Thor—the Norse God of thunder. Some say its symbol is an eagle, and others that it is a lightning bolt or staff.

♄ Saturn is the planet of boundaries, measured/linear time, harvest, control, and all other kinds of limitations. By extension, it is also associated with death, binding, sleep, and darkness. Its color is black, and its metal is lead. Saturn's symbol is the sickle, and its day is, obviously, Saturday.

Planet	Day	Color	Metal	Powers
Moon	Monday	Purple	Silver	Subconscious, Change, Lust
Mercury	Wednesday	Orange	Mercury	Intellect, Pattern, Words
Venus	Friday	Green	Copper	Emotions, Intersubjectivity
Sun	Sunday	Yellow	Gold	Health, Ego, Grace, Vision
Mars	Tuesday	Red	Iron	Conflict, Courage, Strength
Jupiter	Thursday	Blue	Tin	Kingship, Money, Expansion
Saturn	Saturday	Black	Lead	Boundaries, Death, Harvest

MOON

From the position of an earthbound observer, the most striking qualities of the moon are its light and its cycle. Like all luminous beings, the moon is associated with illumination in both literal and metaphorical senses. Lunar deities are often wisdom or knowledge deities. This is particularly true in literate cultures, because it is the moon who taught us humans to write. While archaeological evidence from so deep in prehistory is both scant and difficult to interpret, the earliest records that can be categorized as written appear to be lunar calendars. Such calendars predate anything else we understand as writing by tens of thousands of years and are found all over the world. From these first tally marks, humans first developed written numbers, then pictograms to indicate what was being counted, and these eventually transformed into alphabetic writing as we know it. For this reason, many ancient scribal gods began life as moon gods, and scribing was added to their attributes much later, when writing was invented or imported into their culture of origin. The Egyptian god Thoth is an example of such a lunar scribe god. While this association of the moon and insight/wisdom is very common cross-culturally, it is not an absolute.

Although it is simply not true that all women's cycles align with the moon, there is a significant relationship between the moon's cycle and the menstrual cycle. Many scholars believe that at least some of the lunar calendars I mentioned were actually menstrual calendars. Because of this association, lunar gods often have close ties to female fertility and the women's mysteries. In our culture, the moon is almost always explicitly gendered as female. However, that association is not as universal as you might expect. For example, Thoth is male and has no connection with menstruation that I know of.

Single-Note Incenses for the Moon

All artemisia

Clary sage

Camphor (especially for the dark or new moon)

Jasmine (especially for the full moon)

Most white flowers

Mint

Orris root

Marijuana

Star anise

Incense for the Horned Moon

This incense was originally designed to accompany my coven's performance of a wish-granting rite based on one from the Greek Magical Papyri* that calls upon the Horned Moon. An adaptation of that rite for a single magician follows this recipe. It is excellent for any lunar work, but especially those that deal with the dark, new, or crescent moon, or associated deities, such as Thoth, Hekate, Artemis, or Diana the Huntress. It is especially good for awakening the senses and promoting divinatory trance.

6 parts mugwort

6 parts frankincense

4 parts myrrh

2 parts hyssop

2 parts lemon balm

2 parts star anise

1 part rose petals

1 part dried elderberries

Honey to bind

The Wishing Rite of the Horned Moon

YOU WILL NEED

About an hour during the night of the dark moon, ideally in the hour
   of the moon

A cauldron or Dutch oven filled with about 2 inches of dirt

A candle, in the cauldron

About half a cup of any lunar incense

A cup of heavy cream

---

*   PGM LXX.12.

A white or purple head covering

A black bowl full of water or another scrying surface

It is best to perform this rite outdoors, somewhere dark. Arrange your working space so that you can reach the fire and it glints on your scrying surface. Before beginning, prepare a written petition carefully outlining your request. Any sort of request is okay, but those related to insight, intuition, divination, sex, and psychism are especially appropriate for this work. Write your petition in purple ink on a piece of paper. Soak the paper in amber oil, then blot it off so it's no longer dripping. Fold it into a small triangle.

WHAT TO DO

♦ Cover your head.

♦ Enter into magical space, time, and consciousness by any method.

♦ Light the candle, and begin the oration:

I call upon you who have all forms and many names,

Double-horned* goddess, Moon, brilliant night-flame.

Your true form is a mystery, known only by the One Who Makes,

Who created the world entire, including your twenty-eight shapes.

IAO** IAO IAO

Your forms complete every figure; they taught us how to count.

You breathe out full flourishing life on every creature's account.

You grow from obscurity into light, a flame from tiny spark.

You withdraw your brilliance, giving space once more to the dark.

[At each companion below, put a pinch of incense into the flames.]

The first companion of your name is silence,

The second a ba-popping sound.

---

* This name refers to the shape of the crescent moon.

** IAO is a gnostic variation of the Hebrew godname יהוה.

The third is groaning,

the fourth is hissing,

the fifth a cry of joy, profound.

The sixth is moaning,

The seventh is barking,

The eighth a bellowing bray,

the ninth the horse's neigh.

the tenth is a musical sound,

the eleventh a howling wind,

With the twelfth, you create the wind,

And the thirteenth is a coercive sound.

The final companion of your holy name is the

Holy decree that emanated forth from perfection.

ASKEI KATASKEI* ERON OREAN IOR MEGA SAMNYER
PHOBANTIA SEMNE!

bark bark bark**

Ereshkigal,*** virgin, bitch, serpent, garland, key, caduceus, golden-sandaled Lady of Tartarus, I have been initiated. I went down below the ground, into the chamber of the Dactyls,**** and I saw things below:

[Throw a pinch of incense into the fire for each one.]

The ox,

The vulture,

---

*   These magic words are so common in ancient spells that the phrase "askei kataskei" was the ancient equivalent to our hocus pocus.
**   Bark like a dog.
***   Ereshkigal, a Sumerian Queen of Hell, is closely syncretized with both Hekate and Persephone.
****   A type of magician-smith-priest in the court of the Great Mother.

The bull,

The beetle,

The falcon,

The crab,

The bitch,

The wolf,

The serpent,

The horse,

The she-goat,

The asp,

The sheep,

The he-goat,

The baboon,

The cat,

The lion,

The leopard,

The field mouse,

The deer,

The shape-changer,

The virgin,

The torch,

The lightning,

The garland,

The caduceus,

The child,

And the key.

I have said your secret names and symbols so that you might hear me,

I pray to you, mistress of the whole world, come and draw near to me!

Hear me, O stable one, O mighty one, O Queen of Witches and Wishes:

[Throw your petition into the flames.]

AFEIBOĒŌ MINTĒR OXAŌ PIZEFYDŌR XANTHAR XADĒROZO MOXTHION EOTNEU FĒRZON AINDĒS

LAXABOŌ PITTŌ

RIFTHAMER ZMOMOXŌLEIE TIĒDRANTEIA OISOZOXABĒDŌFRA

♦ Now, drape your headscarf so that you can see nothing but the bowl. Stare into it to see visions from the goddess. When you are done speaking with her, cover the scrying bowl with the headscarf, and return to mundane time, space, and consciousness.

MERCURY

Mercury is the smallest and innermost planet of our solar system. It moves very quickly, completing a circuit around the sun every eighty-eight days. Because it is so fleet, it is often syncretized with travel gods such as the Roman Mercury, the Greek Hermes, and the Babylonian Nabu; however, it has been syncretized with many other gods as well. For example, in ancient Greece, the planet Mercury was often understood as two different bodies, one appearing by morning and sacred to Apollo and another in the evenings sacred to Hermes. In prehistory, most people never traveled very far. Among those that did were messengers, storytellers, translators, and traders. Thus, all of these activities fall naturally into the sphere of Mercury. Additionally, all activities done by one's wits, including literacy, mathematics, fast talk, gambling, conning, sleight of hand, sorcery, spirit-speaking, spirit-travel, and all types of navigating, both literal and metaphoric, belong to the sphere of Mercury.

Mercury does not have a single clear color attribution, but dark purple, bright orange, all neon colors, and rainbow opalescence are all associated with this planet. Some of Mercury's special sacred numbers are 8, 23, 64, 88, and 260; others are 10^{100} (called a googol), $(1\pm\sqrt{5})/2$ (often called the "golden ratio"), and 0. In truth, *all* numbers, and the very concept of number itself, are sacred to Mercury.

This incense was originally designed as an offering to Hermes the Quicksilver King, a modern incarnation of Hermes with whom I partner for work related to eloquence, quick-wittedness, charisma, and the gift of gab. It is an excellent offering for nearly any spirit of the sphere of Mercury and also good as a mood-setting incense for any activity that would benefit from mental sizzle, including writing, math, and teaching. It can also be ground fine and steeped in. It is an especially good choice for market-related magics, whether as seller, buyer, bookkeeper, or thief.

Single-Note Incenses for Mercury

Because of Mercury's role as the traveler/trader of the planets, any incense with a history as a trade good makes a good offering to Mercury. This is especially true if you bought it while traveling. Chios mastic, storax, and amber are especially nice, as is frankincense. Sandalwood, lemongrass, anise, fennel, nutmeg, cloves, marjoram, and saffron are all also classically associated with Mercury. Many people would list lavender here as well. Personally, I like tobacco for Mercury, but many people associate it with Mars.

Mercury Incense Recipe:

> 8 parts frankincense or any other resin for its celestial resonance and its association with travel and trade
>
> 4 parts cedar or any other aromatic wood to focus the mind, transform desire, and evoke a lush, rich, warm feeling
>
> 2 parts cloves for harmony, purity, and especially to draw good luck
>
> 2 parts nutmeg to open the psychic senses
>
> 1 part cinnamon or cassia to get things moving quickly
>
> Honey to bind
>
> 1 strand saffron per burn (Saffron in particular, and crocuses in general, are sacred to Hermes.)

VENUS

Venus's is the sphere of love in its broadest sense; the planet controls all the forces that unite humans one with the other, romance and family, community and communion. Venus's magic is one of the most widely and practically applicable. Anytime you want someone to like you, whether a boss or a neighbor, a mother-in-law or a potential lover, the spirits of the sphere of Venus are the ones you want on your side. If you need help navigating complicated social situations, Venus, the Wile-Weaver, the Charming One, is your greatest ally. All social interconnection between human beings is of the sphere of Venus. But Venus is even more than that; it is the generative force that brings forth life from life.

Venus is the Great Green Goddess. The oldest known use of the name Venus is in the context of the ancient pre-Roman Latin festival of Vinalia Rustica, the celebration of the ripening of the vines and gardens, celebrated in late August. That festival was originally dedicated to Venus Obsequia, Venus the Gracious and Giving. As Latin cultures became Roman ones, the festival was given to Jupiter. Similarly, our cultural understanding of Venus has also been given over to the patriarch. Venus, as we know her today, is much reduced.

Venus is the goddess who taught us to garden, who taught us the relationship between seed and plant. Venus is the goddess of fecundity: the fertile vigor of the garden and the orchard, the field, the livestock, the mother, the community. Venus is the overflowing Greenness of Life, the essential "life-ness" of the soul, *viriditas*. Says Saint Hildegard of Bingen: "There is a power that has been since all eternity and that force and potentiality is green!"

Because the planet orbits between us and the sun, Venus cannot always be seen from Earth. It often disappears on one horizon and reappears on the other. For this reason, some cultures speak of it as two distinct entities; the Evening Star and the Morning Star. However, by the time writing became widespread in Mesopotamia and we have sufficient records to judge, those are known to be the same object. There, it was known by many names: Inanna, Ninsi'anna, the Bright Lady, the Shining One of Heaven, She of Red Skies, the Holy Queen of Heaven and Earth. Most Western cultures, including our own, inherit at least part of their understanding of Venus from this tradition, and it is well worth your time to learn the myths and names. Of them, my favorite text is the Nin Me Šara or "Exaltation of the Goddess," one of the most ancient human sacred texts. Written in the 23rd century BCE by Enheduanna, high priestess of Ur and daughter of the king Sargon of Akkad, Nin Me Šara positions Ishtar as a powerful and politically important goddess of both love and war.

The symbol of the planet Venus, which has become the symbol for femaleness, is usually understood as a hand mirror. In the ancient world, mirrors were often made of copper, Venus's metal. Most ancient Greek copper came from Cyprus, the island of Aphrodite, a Greek goddess associated with Venus. In fact, our English word *copper* is closely related to the name of Cyprus, the copper island. However, the symbol is also linked to the rod and ring symbol of Mesopotamian kingship, very often held by depictions of Inanna and other Mesopotamian Venus goddesses. In Egypt, this same sign was called the shen ring and represented eternal protection. It may also be related to the so-called knot of Isis, also called the *tyet*, which is thought by many to represent a tampon. Others think it may represent a sistrum or a necklace.

In Hermetic systems, Venus's number is seven, and its day is Friday. The goddess is associated with lions, doves, wolves, and peacocks. As mentioned before, its metal is copper, and its gem is the emerald. The angel most often associated with Venus is Anael (לאינה), whose name means "Joy of El," sometimes spelled Haniel.

Single-Note Incenses for Venus

Rose, dittany of Crete, sandalwood, vanilla, most fruits (especially wet ones), most flowers (especially red ones), and most femme perfumes are excellent for the sphere of Venus and all associated spirits.

Offering Incense for the Spirits of Venus

In addition to being used as an offering, this incense can be used to set the mood for love. I also really like to pass jewelry through this smoke to charge it for glamour and beauty.

> 3 parts rose petals (Rose petals given as a gift from lover to lover are
> especially good. Red is my preferred color for this spell.)
> 3 parts pine or another resin (Chios mastic is especially nice.)

2 parts dittany of Crete, awakened as Έρωντας (Erontas)

1 part orange peel

Honey to bind

If you grind everything very fine, and add enough honey to make a paste, this is an excellent beautifying mask for the face. If you exchange the resin for powdered milk and/or salt, this also makes a lovely bath. Grind the herbs very fine, or use a muslin bag, because otherwise it will make a mess in your bathtub.

SUN

The Sun is the center of our solar system, the axis around which the classical planets turn. It stands at the border between the inner, more personal planets—Moon, Mercury, and Venus—and the external/civic ones—Mars, Jupiter, and Saturn. Similarly, the Sun works at those places where our secret inner selves meet the communal outer world. The Sun rules over our sense of identity. The Sun is the source of almost all energy on Earth. Sunlight illuminates, warms, and heals, but it also disinfects, bakes, and burns. Upper World spirits of the Sun are too numerous to list, so I'll just choose a few of my favorites to give you a feel for that variety. As you read through, notice how a culture's sun gods are largely informed by their weather. In the cold, the Sun is all-beneficent and rites surrounding those gods tend to be invocational. On the other hand, desert sun gods are more wrathful, and their rites are often aimed at propitiation to quell its more destructive power.

Helios (Ήέλιος) is the Greek god of the sun. Like his sisters Selene (Moon) and Eos (Dawn), Helios is the child of the Titaness Euryphaessa, the goddess of heavenly bodies, and Hyperion, the Great God. Hyperion and Helios were often syncretized and are difficult to disambiguate. Although sun worship appears to have been widespread in prehistoric Greece, Helios did not have a widespread cult in classical Greece. At that time, his worship was centered on the island of Rhodes, where he was an important tutelary deity. His statue, the Colossus of Rhodes, was one of the Wonders of the World. He rose once more to glory in late antiquity, partly owing to his conflation with the Roman Sol. He is most often depicted as a young and beautiful man wearing a golden crown and driving the chariot of the sun. Helios is an important figure in the Greek Magical Papyri, where he is one of the Great Powers, the source of all life. For example, in PGM IV 1596-1715, he is described thus:

> . . . Greatest God, Eternal Lord, World Ruler, who are over the World and under the World, Mighty Ruler of the Sea, rising at Dawn, shining from the East for the Whole World, setting in the West. Come to me, you who arise from the Four Winds, benevolent and lucky Agathos Daimon, for whom the Heavens are the Processional Way. . . . The Earth flourished when You shone forth, and the Plants became fruitful when you laughed; the Animals begat their Young when You permitted. . . . greatest in Heaven, the Shining Helios, giving Light throughout the Whole World. You are the Great Serpent, Leader of all the Gods, who control the Beginning of Egypt and the End of the Whole Inhabited World . . .

Shemesh (also called Shapash), a Canaanite solar goddess, is the daughter of El and Asherah. She is called the Torch of the Gods or the Divine Illuminator. She is a messenger and psychopomp and similar in many ways to Hekate Dadophoros. She is, like many solar gods, an all-seeing eye whose sunbeams witness everything that transpires on Earth. In one story, she descends to the underworld with her sister Anat to rescue Anat's husband Baal. While there, Anat cries a river of tears, which Shemesh laps up, becoming drunk on them. She flies into a fury, unleashing drought and killing heat on the Earth. Among her favorite offerings are sparkling wine and garlands of bay leaves.

Auriel (לְאִירוּא) is an angelic regent of the sun, whose name means "Light of El." Most scholars agree that the specific traditions of the named angels enter Judaism during the Babylonian Captivity, and this is almost certainly the case for Auriel. Auriel is usually identified as male, but sometimes also depicted as female. They are a cherub (a winged lion with a human head), although in the modern day, they are almost always depicted in human or winged-human form. In iconography, they often carry a book or scroll, representing their gifts of illumination, enlightenment, and wisdom. With a fiery sword, they guard the northern gate of Paradise. Auriel is a great lover of humans and can be called to testify on our behalf in the Heavenly Court. It was they who warned Noah of the impending flood.

They and their underlings were the Passover angel(s), who brought death to the Egyptians, while preserving those Hebrews who painted their doors with lamb's blood. Sunday is their day, and among their favorite offerings is poetry.

Single-Note Solar Incenses

All resins, especially frankincense

Cedar

Clover

Lemongrass

Saffron

Rosemary

Cinnamon

Clove

Citrus

Honey

All-Purpose Solar Offering Incense

This incense is an excellent offering for all spirits of the sphere of the sun. It is particularly nice burned on top of a gold-colored coin. When this is done as an offering, I strongly recommend donating the coin directly to someone in need.

This is also good for healing and works to gently soothe grief or other trauma. It is a mild banisher, good for lifting foggy gloom, especially from rooms full of grief or depression. It fills a space with warmth and happiness; burn it during family gatherings. This mix can also be cold infused as a tea. Drink it alone or mixed into chai or black tea. Use cold water and let it steep overnight. Do not brew with hot water, or the frankincense will make a gummy mess.

5 parts frankincense for its solar power

3 parts citrus peel for lightening and brightening (The more varieties you can include, the better.)

2 parts cinnamon chips for warmth, homeyness, and comfort

1 part lemon balm to keep the mixture green, life-giving, and

    non-wrathful

Honey to bind

MARS

Mars, called the Red Planet, is red because its surface is laden with iron oxide (rust). Of all the planets in our solar system, it is, in many ways, the one most like the Earth. In English, the planet is named after the Roman god of war, sharing similar roots with *martial* and *military*. Mars's month is March, its day is Tuesday, its color is red, and its symbol is the spear and shield. It is associated with wolves and bears, as well as cattle and horses.

This planet is associated with all things martial and manly. It is the masculine principle and represents physical strength, mental discipline, and spiritual courage. Mars's energy is virile, powerful, and direct. Mars helps you defend yourself and prove yourself. All ambition belongs to it. Mars is that fortune which favors the bold. Mars gets a bad reputation in our culture, which tends to paint it as an uncivilized brute, just as we tend to portray Venus as a stupid bimbo. Both of these unjust caricatures are reflections of toxic patriarchy. Examine your own beliefs to root them out. Much of the Mars revilement in our culture is inherited from classical Athens, where Ares (the Greek equivalent of Mars) was the patron god of their enemy, Sparta. Almost every Greek story you've ever heard about Ares (or Mars) is at least partly Athenian political propaganda.

Mars magic can help steel you for battle and also aid you in finding calm in the center of chaos. It can be employed to improve confidence before an interview and provides strong and reliable protection. Mars's help is also excellent to attract male sex partners or to ramp up your own sexiness as a man. Mars's martiality is protective and community-minded; it fights to protect home and family, tribe and land. Mars guards the boundaries of the fields, preventing wild nature from creeping back in. Mars is also good for justice work.

For a quick spot of martial protection, repeat "Mars, Māvors, macte est"* under your breath, and imagine an iron fence surrounding you. On top of the

---

*   "Mars Mavors is to be honored." Mavors is an ancient name for Mars.

fence, imagine shadow soldiers in gleaming armor, wearing red cloaks that flutter behind them like Superman's. They leap, cavorting, from fence post to fence post, pounding their spears on their gleaming shields, dancing their warrior dance. Experiment with imagining them going both clockwise and counterclockwise. Experiment with how many there are; I like five.

Single-Note Incenses for Mars

Dragon's blood

Pine

Basil

Wormwood

Allspice

Tobacco

Offering Incense for Mars

This incense is excellent as an offering for all spirits of the sphere of Mars. It can be huffed to invoke martial gods and their prowess and to steel your courage for battle. It's also nice while working out. Thyme, hawthorn, and salt together also make a very nice post-workout bath.

2 parts resin (A mixture of dragon's blood and myrrh is especially good
for this.)

1 part wormwood

1 part thyme

1 part hawthorn

1 part tobacco

JUPITER

Jupiter is the largest of the planets; more than twice as large as all the others put together. I have frequently heard people say that it is almost large enough to have become a second sun, but that is not the case. Jupiter is less than 1/1,000th the size of our Sun, and about 1/75th the size of the smallest stars. That being said, Jupiter is thermally radiant and slowly shrinking. Its surface is covered in roiling clouds and storms the size of continents.

Astrologically, the planet is called the Greater Beneficent and the bringer of miracles. Its power is broadly expansive, growing field and bank account, kingdom and influence. Jupiter can help you be a better father, leader, or judge, and it can help win those people to your side.

The planet Jupiter takes its English name from the Roman god Iupiter, who is one of a coterie of gods with names evolved from Indo-European *Dyēu-pəter ("Father Sky" or "God the Father"). Zeus Pater, for example, is the Greek incarnation. This god is complicated and multifaceted; he is the god of leadership and fatherhood, but also of empire and patriarchy. He is the king of the gods and wields a lightning bolt as his scepter and weapon. He is associated with eagles, bulls, oak trees, thunder, lightning, and mountains. One great and easy token of Jupiter is the old style of U.S. quarter with George Washington (our Father-King) on one side and his eagle on the other.

Single-Note Offerings for Jupiter

Frankincense

Thunderstruck oak

Cedar

Pine (resin or needles or both)

Clove

Hyssop

Rosemary

Incense for the Beneficent King

This incense is excellent as an offering for all spirits of the sphere of Jupiter and can also be used in most Jovial sorcery, including the spell below designed to secure the support of a wealthy and/or powerful patron.

5 parts frankincense or another resin

2 parts juniper or other needles

1 part cedar or another aromatic wood

1 part rosemary

1 part cloves

A Spell to Acquire a Wealthy Patron

This spell is best performed on a Thursday, during the hour of Jupiter, while the moon waxes. However, you can perform it at any time, and then recharge it when the time is right. The goal of the spell is to attract the attention, favor, and patronage of someone wealthy and powerful. While this spell will help grease the wheels, you'll still need to seal the deal with mundane work.

YOU WILL NEED

> A piece of bristol board or another heavy paper
>
> A bowl or something else to trace a circle
>
> Scissors
>
> A pen
>
> A description of the patron you'd like (This can be either by name and/or photo to enchant a particular person or by qualities if you don't have someone specific in mind.)
>
> Six quarters or other coins
>
> Charcoal and a way to light it
>
> About ¼ cup of incense for Jupiter

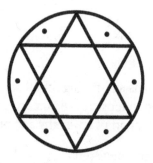

Solomon's Seal

WHAT TO DO

♦ Trace a circle onto the bristol board and cut it out.

- On one side, write the description of your patron. Turn the circle ninety degrees and sign your name over it, entangling them together.

- On the other side of the paper, draw Solomon's seal, like the one above.

- In the interior hexagon, draw the symbol of Jupiter.

- Stack the quarters carefully on top of the Jupiter symbol, and put the lit charcoal on top of them.

- Feed small pieces of incense to the charcoal, while you . . .

- Speak your wish in great detail to the incense. Describe exactly what you want to happen.

- When the charcoal has fully burned down, retrieve the amulet you've drawn on this paper and burn it to ash.

- Mix the ash into the remaining incense, and burn the incense each Thursday for four weeks.

SATURN

Saturn is my favorite of the classical planets. It is the farthest planet, the boundary of the known world. It is the liminal space between one place and another. Saturn, as its name suggests, is satiated. Saturn is death, but also liberation. Saturn is a useful magical ally in any work that involves limiting or containing anything. In English, the planet Saturn is named after the Roman god Saturn, the King of the Golden Age and master of the sickle, which he uses both to bring in the grain and to castrate his abusive father. He is a god of agriculture, civilization and good order, the social contract, and old age. In syncretic late antiquity, the god of Israel was understood to be a face of Saturn, and Saturn-dread and anti-Semitism are tightly wound together in Western culture. This makes Saturn an especially good magical ally for containing and restricting anti-Semitism, white supremacy, and many forms of fascism.

Single-Note Incenses for Saturn

Myrrh

Bergamot

Cypress

Thyme

Offering Incense for the Sphere of Saturn

6 parts myrrh

6 parts mugwort

2 parts thyme

2 parts elderberries

1 part marijuana (optional)

An Oracle of Saturn

INSPIRED BY PGM IV 3086-3124

YOU WILL NEED

A salt grinder and salt

A mirror

Saturn incense, ground to a fine powder and added to olive oil to make a
thin paste

Saturn incense, with added honey (for extra smoke)

WHAT TO DO

◆ Anoint your third eye with the symbol of Saturn, using the oil and
incense paste.

◆ Draw the same sigil on the mirror, filling most of it.

◆ Light the incense and place it between you and the mirror.

◆ Slowly grind salt onto the incense from high above.

- While you do so, say aloud:

I call to you, Great and Holy One, you who created the entire inhabited world. You who were slain by your own son. You whom Helios bound in adamantine fetters. You, hermaphrodite! You, Father of Thunderbolt! You who hold down the Earth.

AIE OI PAIDALIS PHRENOTEICHEIDO

STYGARDE SANKLEON GENECHRONA

KOIRAPSAI KERIDEU THALAMNIA OCHOTA ANEDEI

Come, Lord God, and tell me everything about

————————————————————*.*

None but Kronos, none but he whom I have called may come.

This I command in the names of those who revolted! In the name of mighty Zeus!

PAIDOLIS MAINOLIS MAINOLIEUS

KYDOBRIS KODERIEUS ANKYRIEUS XANTOMOULIS

- Unfocus your eyes and stare at the mirror through the smoke. Rock back and forth, taking your face in and out of the smoke. Speak glossolalia, breathe deeply, and let go until you feel the god arise and begin to answer your question.

- When you are done, say:

ANAEA OCHETA THALAMNIA KERIDEU KOIRAPSI
    GENECHRONA SANELON STYGARDES CHLEIDO
    PHRAINLOE PAIDOLIS IAEL.

Goodbye, master of the world, forefather, go to your own place in the universe, and there be sated. Be gracious, Lord.

Alternatively, the same procedure may be done just before sleep, and the oracle sought in dreams instead of in the mirror.

Offering Incense for the Guardians of the Gates of Outer Darkness

There is a phenomenon that appears strange but is easily understood when you let go of your human preconceptions about what shape the universe ought to be: It is very difficult to distinguish between the regions at the heights of the Upper World and those at the depths of the Lower World. That is to say, once you're sufficiently far away from the Middle World "native habitat" of humans, it becomes increasing difficult to perceive anything at all; eventually, there is only darkness. The universe is not linear; it is only your experience living in a human body that makes you think "up" and "down" are fundamentally incompatible. In these places, furthest from Earth, things exist at scales nigh incomprehensible to humans. This is the primordial soup of cosmic creation, the Tohu wa Bohu of probabilistic complexity from which everything arises and into which everything returns.

1 part frankincense
3 parts juniper
1 part mint
1 part thyme

Offerings for Named Spirits

BECAUSE NEARLY ALL spirits make their homes in at least one of the Three Worlds we discussed in the previous chapter, we can now use those recipes as a basis for expansion, adapting and mixing them to create signature blends for any particular spirit. In this chapter, we'll see several examples of different ways to create such individualized recipes. I've simply chosen some of my favorite spirits to use as examples; I encourage you to experiment with creating your own blends for your best beloved spirits.

Hekate: Queen of Witches

Hekate is the goddess of magic and gateways, ghosts and crossroads. As the goddess of sorcery and initiation, every liminal space is hers; she is the gatekeeper of every mystery. Throughout the classical world, shrines and statues of Hekate were placed by gateways, the gates of cities and temples, as well as the doors of individual homes. In addition to her role guarding literal doorways, Hekate is also a goddess of the threshold between our world and the Other Place. In mythology both classical and modern, Hekate is unquestionably an initiator of all who seek to travel between the worlds. Hekate is the Queen of Witches; she teaches magic to those who seek her wisdom. This is the role I've sought to capture in this incense: Hekate as an initiatrix and gate-opener.

> 3 parts mugwort for its connection with Artemis, the moon, necromancy,
> and witchcraft

2 parts dittany of Crete for its ability to aid trance and time travel

3 parts frankincense for Hekate's shining crown of starlight

1 part Chios mastic for the lightness of her youth and the depths of the
cerulean Aegean

Marijuana "to taste"

Honey to bind

This incense is an excellent offering to Hekate, as well to other spirits associated with witchcraft. It's mildly trance-inducing and a good choice for almost any witchcraft, particularly lunar or saturnian work. As usual, you should awaken each ingredient to its virtues before mixing, and then bless the whole mixture when it is complete. For this incense, I like to bless with the following rite, best performed on a new moon, which is adapted from PGM IV 2708-2784.

> *O Hekate of many names, O Virgin, Kore,* * *Goddess, come, I ask,*
>
> *O guard and shelter of the threshing floor, Persephone,*
>
> *O triple-headed goddess, who walks on fire,*
>
> *cow-eyed BOUORPHORBÊ*
>
> *PANPHORBA*
>
> *PHORBARA*
>
> *AKTIÔPHI*
>
> *ERESCHIGAL*
>
> *NEBOUTOSOUALÊTH beside the doors,*
>
> *PYPYLÊDEDEZÔ and gate-breaker;*
>
> *Come, Hekate, of fiery counsel, I call you to my sacred chants.*
>
> *MASKELLI MASKELLÔ*
>
> *PHNOUKENTABAÔTH*

---

*   This is the Greek word for "maiden" or "adult woman without children." It is a title that applies to many goddesses, particularly Persephone.

OREOBAZAGRA who burst forth from the earth

OREOPÊGANYX MORMORON TOKOUMBAI!

Hekate, I have called to you by your ancient names of power.

Come be with me, and speak to me, and bless your holy incense.

Come be with me, and speak to me, and bless your holy incense.

Authors & Teachers of the Greek Magical Papyri

As you've doubtless put together by now, I am particularly fond of a collection of ancient spell books called the Papyri Graecae Magicae (Greek Magical Papyri), or PGM. The texts were written in Greek-speaking Egypt in late antiquity, mostly dating between 200 BCE and 400 CE. They were translated into English by a collective of scholars, led by Hans Dieter Betz, at the University of Chicago. The works in the PGM were not collected together in antiquity; they represent only snapshots into a huge and largely unknown corpus, the lone survivors of centuries of both Christian and Muslim destruction of magical texts.

Close reading of the collection makes it very clear that the authors were quite diverse. Some appear to be well-educated and privileged members of the Egyptian priesthood primarily concerned with mystic and spiritual development. Others appear to be professional village witches, who worked results-oriented magic for their communities. Some use Greek god names, some Egyptian, some Hebrew, and some unidentifiable. Most use a combination of all of these. In my own studies of the PGM, I found myself wanting to offer thanks to the people who invented, wrote, taught, and preserved these spells and to seek their aid in my own magical work. I made this incense for them.

There are several kinds of incense mentioned in the PGM: frankincense, rose, heliotrope, myrrh, myrtle, storax, bay, lotus, spikenard, cinnamon, saffron, and many others. Additionally, several recipes for different incenses are given. Additionally, we know several traditional incense recipes from the cultures that come together in the PGM, kyphi and ketoret in particular. For this reason, I wanted to include many of these ingredients and scent profiles. However, I didn't want an incense for working magic from the PGM. I wanted an incense to offer not to the spirits honored in the PGM, but the spirits of the humans who wrote, practiced, and taught this magic. For this reason, I started with the Mighty Dead offering incense as a starting point.

Since cloves are not common in the PGM, but cinnamon is, I began by making that change. Next, I added some wormwood, noted for aiding in communication with the dead, to help strengthen the evocation. The authors of the PGM are a misty group, not well remembered, and so they need more support than better-known Mighty Dead. For a similar reason, and because myrrh is such a powerful spirit in the PGM, I changed half the frankincense to myrrh. However, I didn't want the mixture to be too dark from the wormwood and myrrh, so I added some bright, solar bay. Not only does the bay balance the more chthonic elements, but it was also used for visionary work in both Greece and Egypt. After making several test batches, these are the proportions I like best, but as we've discussed before, the best proportions will vary in each batch, because natural ingredients are not consistent between gatherings.

>   3 parts frankincense
>
>   3 parts myrrh
>
>   2 parts cedar
>
>   1 part cinnamon
>
>   1 part bay
>
>   1 part rose
>
>   1 part dittany of Crete
>
>   Honey to bind

Solomon, the Magician King

King Solomon is my favorite of the biblical Mighty Dead. I work with him as a tribal ancestor as well as a beloved teacher. Solomon, son of David, is one of the great figures in Jewish mytho-history. If you don't know much about him, you should learn more. He is widely regarded not just by Jews, but by Muslims, Christians, and Near Eastern Pagans as well, as an embodiment of wisdom and magic. He built the great Temple of Jerusalem and mastered the free djinn. He spoke the languages of all the animals and wrote the grimoires. He is the archetype of the magician king.

With this incense, I invoke Solomon as a preliminary practice before so-called Solomonic-style magic, and I also seek wisdom from him in my dreams. This incense is not the incense offered in Solomon's Temple, called ketoret. You will find a recipe for ketoret in the final chapter of this book.

KING SOLOMON OFFERING INCENSE

3 parts frankincense for kingship and worldly power

2 parts myrrh for power in the Underworld and among the dead

1 part cedarwood for the great pillars of the Temple, the great Ashera
world tree

1 part cedar needles for the gentleness of the wind in the needles of the
trees that gave strength of the pillars

1 part cinnamon for its rich and costly perfume and for its warmth

1 part rose petals for love, beauty, and luxury

THE INVOCATION OF SOLOMON

This invocation of Solomon is a good preparation for any type of Solomonic magic. Like most preparatory invocations, it is designed to allow the magician to speak magic in the name of the power—in this case Solomon—being invoked.

It is presented in two versions. The first is for Jews, Ethiopians, and others who have an ancestral connection to Solomon. The other is for people who do not. I have done this so you can see examples of how to frame practices for both your own tribal ancestors and more universal Mighty Dead like saints and folk heroes. Notice that in the first version, the identification with Solomon is as an ancestor, and the claim being made is that Solomon's authority is inheritable. In the second, we draw on his power as a religious figure and establish the intimacy by highlighting spiritual similarities between ourselves and Solomon. Both invocations largely parallel the עץ חיים (Etz Chaim), or Tree of Life. The first version is a relatively straightforward ascent from bottom to top, very loosely modeled on *Pardes Rimonim*, a classic text by the16th-century kabbalist Moshe ben Jakov

Cordovero. The second is only slightly modified from the 19th-century Christian magician Eliphas Levi's *Dogme et Rituel de la Haute Magie*.

Version One

> *I am NAME, inheritor of the line of Abraham, blood kin to Solomon the King. My blood is his blood, and his kingdom is mine. I invoke Solomon, djinn master, temple builder. I invoke Solomon, the magician and the king.*

> *I am NAME, inheritor of the line of Isaac, blood kin to Solomon the King. My blood is his blood, and his foundation is mine. I invoke Solomon, djinn master, temple builder. I invoke Solomon, the magician and the king.*

> *I am NAME, child of the house of Jakob, blood kin to Solomon the King. My blood is his blood, and his brilliance is mine. I invoke Solomon, djinn master, temple builder. I invoke Solomon, the magician and the king.*

> *I am NAME, child of mother Leah, blood kin to Solomon the King. My blood is her blood, and her victory is mine. I invoke Solomon, djinn master, temple builder. I invoke Solomon, the magician and the king.*

> *I am NAME, child of mother Rachel, blood kin to Solomon the King. My blood is her blood, and her beauty is mine. I invoke Solomon, djinn master, temple builder. I invoke Solomon, the magician and the king.*

> *I am NAME, inheritor of the line of Rebekah, blood kin to Solomon the King. My blood is her blood, and her power is mine. I invoke Solomon, djinn master, temple builder. I invoke Solomon, the magician and the king.*

> *I am NAME, inheritor of the line of Sarah, blood kin to Solomon the King. My blood is her blood, and her glory is mine. I invoke Solomon, djinn master, temple builder. I invoke Solomon, the magician and the king.*

Repeat the invocation "I invoke Solomon, djinn mastr, temple builder. I invoke Solomon, the magician and the king," over and over at increasing tempo and volume until you feel the power crescendo and you are confident in your ability to command spirits in the name of, and with the full authority of, Solomon the Magician King.

Version Two

> *Like Solomon, the powers of the Kingdom are under my feet and in my hands.*

> *Like Solomon, Glory and Eternity take me by the shoulders and direct me in the paths of victory.*

> *Like Solomon, in Mercy and Justice, I find the equilibrium of my life.*

> *Like Solomon, I am crowned in Intelligence and Wisdom.*

> *Spirits of the Kingdom, lead me between the two pillars on which rest the whole edifice of the temple.*

> *Angels of Victory and Brilliance, establish me on the cubic stone Foundation.*

> *Angels, be with me now as I do this work, be my strength and my love, my brethren in battle.*

> *Creatures of Holiness, cry, speak, roar, bellow!*

> *Holy, Holy, Holy!*

> *Solomon, master of angels and demons and all he surveys, be with me now as I speak in your name!*

Tzadkiel, Angel of the Violet Flame

Tzadkiel (לאיקדצ), the angel of tzedek, is the archangel most often associated with the sphere of Jupiter. He is a leader of the order of angels called the Hashmallim, or Dominions. The word *tzedek*, in Hebrew, means "righteous person" or "saint" and is also the name of the planet Jupiter, the Righteous King. Tzedekah (הקדצ) is an important concept in Jewish mysticism and one that cannot be captured by any single English word. It is often translated as "mercy" or "charity," although almost no one actually thinks those are good translations. In most contexts, the word means more like "justice" or "righteousness," although even those fail to capture its full meaning. I like to think of tzedekah more broadly as "right action" or "action in accord with Creation." Legendarily, Tzadkiel is the angel who held back Abraham's hand when Isaac lay bound before him. He is sometimes called the Angel of the Violet Flame, and under this name he bears the message that we are all called to the ongoing work of creation. Below is a simple method for invoking the presence of Tzadkiel and an accompanying incense. Both are easily modified for any angel.

OFFERING INCENSE FOR TZADKIEL

To develop an incense for a particular angel, we'll start with our basic Upper World recipe and then personalize it. This is that base recipe:

4 parts mixed resins

2 parts rose or another sweet flower

1 part cedar or another aromatic wood

Honey to bind

For this particular recipe, I switched the rose out for hyssop, because I wanted to give it a slightly more delicate and ethereal smell. Additionally, hyssop, with its blue flowers, is an excellent choice for spirits of the sphere of Jupiter, like Tzadkiel. In order to increase the Jupiter vibe and to play up the color of the flowers, I added 1 part juniper berries. Since I already had the pale blue of the hyssop and the dark indigo of the berries, I chose to include violets, largely for their color, but also because wildflowers are always appropriate for angels.

That gives a final recipe of:

4 parts resin

1 part cedar

1 part hyssop

1 part violets

1 part juniper berries

Honey to bind

TO SEEK CONVERSATION WITH AN ANGEL

Arrange a mirror so it reflects the light of a white candle through the smoke of the incense. Have at hand a good supply of clean, unlined white paper and several black ink pens. You may also wish to have colored pens handy.

Make sure you are clear of mind and clean of spirit. Enter magical space, time, and consciousness by any method. The invocation of Solomon above is one good choice. Prayer is especially appropriate for angelic invocation. Take the pen in your hand, poised over the paper, and recite something like the following in your best magician voice:

> O you glorious and benevolent angel, Tzadkiel, Tzadkiel, Tzadkiel, angel of the violet flame, angel of the sphere of Jupiter, I invoke you, adjure you, and call you forth to visible apparition in and through the great and divine Name of the Most High G-d, El Chai,* El Shaddai,** who is Elohim v'Daat,*** and by the ineffable and efficacious virtues and powers thereof, whereby you are governed and called forth, it being absolutely necessary, and ordained, appointed and decreed, and by the obeisance you have made, I do most earnestly entreat and powerfully command you, O you benign angel Tzadkiel, angel of the sphere of Jupiter, come to me now.
>
> I command you, Tzadkiel, to move and appear to me visibly and audibly in this mirror here before me. In and through this same mirror, transmit your ray to my sight, and your voice to my ears, that I might hear you and plainly see you. Move my hand that I might see your writing, and transmit to me your revelation and your sign. Include me in your mysteries, that I might be the instrument of the Most High. I earnestly adjure you, O benevolent and amicable angel, Tzadkiel, in the most excellent Name of G-d, Adonai**** Elohim, I am the servant

---

*   God of Life

**   *Shaddai* is difficult to translate. It is related to the words for demons, mountains, and breasts. El Shaddai is generally understood to the be the God of Sexual Reproduction as a force driving evolution on Earth.

***   God(s) of Knowledge

****   Lord or Master

of the Name, and by the Name I conjure you; show yourself firmly to me, and let me partake of your wisdom. Tzadkiel, Tzadkiel, Tzadkiel, I invoke you now. Tzadkiel, Tzadkiel, Tzadkiel, I invoke you now. . . .

Continue to repeat "Tzadkiel, Tzadkiel . . . now!" until he makes his presence known. If you don't feel anything, start writing the invocation while you read it, and don't stop writing. When you get to the end of the invocation, just keep writing, even if it's just a list of free word associations. As the presence makes itself known, you will begin to engage in what is known as automatic writing, where the angel will write through you, giving you some sort of revelation or message. Feel free to modify the invocation to better suit your own style. You will see several other styles over the course of the book. The worst thing that will happen is nothing.

Asklepios Incense

Asklepios, whose name is closely related to the English word *scalpel,* is a Greek god of healing. He is a son of Apollo, the god of light, and foster son of Chiron, the best of all the centaurs. Snake, the great wisdom-teacher, is his close companion. As a child, Asklepios's ears were licked clean by serpents. From that point on, he could understand the language of the plants and animals, of the winds and the mountains, of Sky, Earth, and Sea. From Chiron, he learned medicine, including the art of surgery. From his father, he learned the arts of prophecy. His temples, the Asklepia, were hospitals as well as centers for dream incubation. If you had an ailment your own village healer couldn't cure, you came to one of the great Asklepia to seek treatment. There, in underground chambers, patients were taught how to seek healing instruction in their dreams. During the night, the god would come and tell them what they must do to get better and also instruct the doctor-priests.

There were many, many Asklepia in the Greek world, but perhaps the most famous were those at Epidaurus, Kos, and Pergamum. Epidaurus, in the Peloponnese, is famed as the first Asklepion, the home of Asklepios when he was still a mortal man. Near to the Asklepion of Epidaurus is the great Theater of Dionysus. I have been taught that, in ancient days, there was always a theater near each Asklepion. Asklepios's surgery is medicine for the body; Dionysus's theater is medicine for the soul.

The Asklepion of Kos, in the Dodecanese, was connected to the great medical school of Hippocrates, the father of what we now call "Western medicine." Here "modern" and "traditional" medicine operated together. The Asklepion of Pergamum, in modern Turkey, home of the physician Galen, specialized in what we would now call mental health and was built around sacred healing springs.

    3 parts frankincense for the healing vitality of the sun

    2 parts bay as the scalpel of Apollo

    1 part dittany of Crete for healing

    1 part thyme for purification

    Honey to bind and also make the medicine go down

Incense for the Great Lioness

Originally designed for the Egyptian goddess Sekhmet, this blend is good for all lion-form goddesses, all goddesses who drive a chariot drawn by lions, and most red goddesses. With this incense, I wanted to show you how to tell a story with the ingredients.

Ra, the shining sun, the king of the gods, grew old and feeble.

The humans mocked him, respecting him not.

Sekhmet, who loved Ra, grew angry.

She stalked the desert mad with rage.

She spilled the blood of many in her anger.

But the clever one, Thoth, knew what to do!

They dyed the beer red, like blood, and fed it to the lion goddess.

And she lapped up the beer, rivers of beer, oceans of beer, until she was sated.

And fell back to sleep, happy and content.

1 part orange peel for the fast-fading glory of the summer sun

1 part garlic peels for the shame we should feel over how we treat our
  elders

1 part cinnamon for Sekhmet's fierce love of Ra

1 part rosemary needles for the sharp claws of her anger

2 parts frankincense, ground fine, for the hot desert sands

3 parts rose petals for the blood poured out

1 part cloves for clever Thoth's pen

1 part hops flower for the beer with which she is sated

Honey to bind all together in sweetness

The Great Bear

A hot topic of debate among scholars for generations, the existence of a pan-European paleolithic bear cult—remnants of which remain to this day—is a deeply inspiring idea for me. While I am unconvinced that there was a single widespread practice, what is unquestionable is the existence of a great number of bear cults all over the world, some existing to this day, and so I assume that there must have been some paleolithic bear cults as well. Below the incense recipe, you'll find a ritual of initiation into an apocryphal cult of the Great Bear Mother, who is also Ursa Major.

3 parts mugwort for its relationship to Artemis, especially in her
  bear form

3 parts juniper needles for the magic of the frigid north gate

1 part cedar for the World Tree, the mighty axis around which the
  Great Bear circles

1 part dried crab apples or another fruit for the bounty and beauty of
  the forest

INITIATION INTO THE CULT OF
THE GREAT BEAR MOTHER

VERY LOOSELY BASED ON PGM VII 686-782

YOU WILL NEED

The incense above or a similar blend

A bear mask

Red ocher in fat (Bear fat is ideal, but ghee, coconut oil, or something similar is also okay.)

An offering for the Great Bear that you can also eat (Berries, nuts, and honey are a nice choice. Planting a blueberry bush or another berry native to you is also a great offering, but be sure there's food as well. You'll also need cool, clean water.)

Recorded drum sounds and a way to play them (You can't drum yourself, because you need both hands free.)

About an hour of free time, ideally late night when the moon is full and the sky is clear

I have only ever performed this in the north, where Ursa Major is always in the sky. If you are in the Southern Hemisphere, this might not be the initiation for you, but you're welcome to experiment with it. I recommend practicing the invocation several times before beginning. You don't need to get it perfectly word for word, but you can't read it during the ritual, because you'll be mostly Bear by then, and Bear can't read.

Before beginning, strip naked, and draw spirals, chevrons, and other paleolithic-seeming patterns on your skin with the red ocher fat. If possible, go out under the moon naked. If not, put a robe on before going out. If you must stay inside, that's okay, but very far from ideal. If possible, when indoors, perform the ritual in a basement or other space under the earth. Light the incense. Ideally, make a small campfire, and throw the incense in it as the ritual progresses. Begin the drum sounds. Put on your mask. Dance as a Bear. Dance until you are sure you are mostly Bear. Look up at the moon, and say something inspired by . . .

Bear, Bear, you who rule the heavens, the stars, and the entire world; you who make the axis turn, you who control the whole cosmos by only force and will, I appeal to you, imploring and supplicating that you accept me into your cult and coterie. Bring me into the Circle Deep, the well of my most ancient ancestors. Do this thing because I call upon you by all your holy names, at which your divinity rejoices, which you cannot ignore. BRIMO, Earth-Breaker, Queen of the Hunt, BAUBO . . . AMOR AMOR AMOR, IEA, shooter of deer AMAM AMAR APHROU, All Queen, Wish Queen, AMAMA, well-bedded, Dardanian, all-seeing, night-running, man-attacker, man-subduer, man-summoner, man-conqueror, LICHRISSA PHAESSA, O ethereal one, O strong one, O lover of song and dance, protectress, spy, delight, delicate, protector, adamant, adamantine, O Damnameneia, BREXERIKANDARA, most high Taurian, unutterable, fire-bodied, light-giving, sharply armed. Admit me into your cult, accept me into the Circle Deep.

And then go right back to dancing. Dance, feeling that this ritual or something similar was performed by your ancient, ancient ancestors. Tens of thousands of years of footbeats whisper around you. The ancestors are coming to join you! Dance, dance, dance, Great Bear, and feel all the others dance with you. When you cannot dance anymore, when you are a tired bear, eat half the offering, drink some water, and go to sleep to dream bearish dreams. You'll be human again when you wake up.

Johnny Appleseed

On the autumnal equinox, in the year 1774, John Chapman was born in Leominster, Massachusetts. When he came of age, Johnny walked west, wandering. That was the year 1792. He walked south, and he walked west. We don't know exactly which way he wandered, but when the Whiskey Rebellion broke out two years later, Johnny Chapman was here in Pittsburgh. He had an orchard out on Grant's Hill, where now stands Mellon Square. He was a cider-maker, and a liquoring man, and he fought against President Washington; he fought for liberty. Here, among the violence and struggle of the Whiskey Rebellion, Johnny heard the call that would turn him into a saint, and it came in a strange form. "Go west," said the voice. "Spread my word," said the voice. "Plant my seeds," said the voice. "Go west."

And so Johnny gathered up his best apples, seeds, his most treasured possessions, and his best cooking pot, which he wore like a cap over his long flowing hair. He gave away his orchard, and he began to walk west.

After he'd walked a spell, he planted his seeds, and he built himself a little cabin, and he began to preach his gospel. "Love your neighbor," he taught. "Love the Earth," he taught. "Be generous, be kind, and forgive." So says the legend: when asked why he feared neither man nor beast, he replied that he lived in harmony with all people and all living things, and that he could not be harmed as long as he lived by the law of love. Johnny Appleseed would not even graft his trees, because he thought it made the trees suffer.

Along with apple seeds, he is said to have sown the seeds of medicinal herbs wherever he went: fennel, pennyroyal, catnip, hoarhound, mullein, rattlesnake root, and more. He healed the sick, when he could, with his herbal potions, and he taught his recipes to any who wanted to learn. Everywhere he went, he learned about their plants and their healing ways, and those too he spread far and wide. He taught people how to make cider. He charged six cents a seedling for apple trees, but only for those that could afford it. For those that couldn't, he would take a bit of cast-off clothing, a bit of food, a story, or nothing at all, from each according to what they could give.

And then, after a few years, when the new trees set fruit, he would gather the very best seeds, and he would give away his cottage and his orchard, and he would set to wandering again. He wandered all over, heading west, planting trees, teaching the truth, as best he knew it. He did no harm to any person, nor even to any beast. When he heard of a horse gone lame, that a farmer would kill, he bought it and set it free to heal. He rescued a wolf cub from a trap, and that wolf followed him all of his days. Barefoot he wandered, over snow and ice. It was said the skin on his feet was so thick, it might kill a rattlesnake if it even tried to bite him. But none ever did. Johnny Appleseed loved the Land, and the Land loved him back. Fifty years or more he wandered, until he came to rest in March of 1845 near Fort Wayne, Indiana.

When Prohibition came, the FBI cut down most of the orchards Johnny Appleseed had planted, because they were used to make cider, the people's drink. And yet, the spirit of Johnny Appleseed lives on, teaching healing, generosity, peacemaking, and the wisdom of Apple.

INCENSE FOR JOHNNY APPLESEED

Although Johnny Appleseed rejoices among the Mighty Dead, he is primarily a spirit of the Middle World and of his beloved Apple Tree. This recipe is designed primarily to highlight the apple, while surrounding it with healing native plants. If Johnny Appleseed lives in your region, so do all these plants.

> 1 part dried apples or crab apples
>
> 3 parts apple blossoms
>
> 1 part applewood
>
> 2 parts pine resin
>
> 1 part blue vervain
>
> 1 part white clover flower
>
> 1 part spicebush
>
> 1 part tobacco (optional)

That Shrewd and Knavish Sprite

At his root, Puck is a British fairy spirit. While originally the name *puck* was for a class of spirits, Shakespeare's characterization of one Puck in *A Midsummer Night's Dream* cemented his identity as a particular, clever faerie, both devious and helpful, mischievous and lucky.

> *That shrewd and knavish sprite*
>
> *Call'd Robin Goodfellow: are not you he*
>
> *That frights the maidens of the villagery;*
>
> *Skim milk, and sometimes labour in the quern*
>
> *And bootless make the breathless housewife churn;*
>
> *And sometime make the drink to bear no barm;*
>
> *Mislead night-wanderers, laughing at their harm?*
>
> *Those that Hobgoblin call you and sweet Puck,*
>
> *You do their work, and they shall have good luck:*
>
> *Are not you he?*

This reputation is underlined in "The Mad Merry Pranks of Robin Goodfellow":

From Oberon in fairyland,

the king of ghosts and shadows there,

Mad Robbin I, at his command,

am sent to view the night sports here:

What revell rout

Is kept about,

In every corner where I goe,

I will o'er see,

And merry be,

And make good sport with ho, ho, ho!

For many, our image of Puck comes primarily, if not directly, from Rudyard Kipling's "Puck of Pook's Hill." In that book, Puck, "the oldest Old Thing in England," appears as "a small, brown, broad-shouldered, pointy-eared person with a snub nose, slanting blue eyes, and a grin that ran right across his freckled face."

The incense recipe below was formulated as an offering for Puck, but with very minor adaptations, it could be used for almost any nature or crossroads spirit.

> 3 parts resin for the eternally shining sun and her infinite bounty
>
> 3 parts apple blossoms for the newness of the spring
>
> 1 part mugwort for the dark places under the hills
>
> 1 part spicebush to give it a little trickster kick
>
> 1 part amanita because what's a fairy incense without toadstools?

Spellwork with Incense

PERSONALLY, MY FAVORITE way to use incense is as the basis for spell-work. However, I want to take one more opportunity to remind you that the division between mood setting, devotional offering, and spellwork is relatively arbitrary. Almost every incense in the book can be used for all three purposes. Similarly, the divisions between types of spellwork in this chapter are quite flexible; they are intended only to serve as a scaffolding for learning. As with every recipe in the book, I encourage you to use these recipes and spells as examples to inspire you to create your own. I have tried to provide a variety of types and sources, to offer a sort of smorgasbord of magical techniques to experiment with.

Divination & Trance

Divination is an art of coming to know things, and to a lesser extent the art of communicating known things to others. It is a broad category of methods to learn and teach. What distinguishes divination from other forms of knowing is that it is inspired. That is to say, it occurs by the action of a non-normal spirit inside us; we are in-spirit-ed. Being good at divination means you can know things you're not supposed to know; a good diviner is dependably a very good guesser. There are several skills involved in divination. While the incenses in this chapter will primarily support magic skills for divination, such as clearing the mind, honing the senses, and attaining and holding deep but navigable trance, far more important than these skills are the mundane ones of paying careful and sustained attention, broad-view pattern recognition, and asking clear, precise questions.

LIBANOMANCY

There are several traditional methods for divining Truth by incense smoke; broadly such techniques are called libanomancy. The word *libanomancy* is based on the Greek λίβανος (*libanos*), which means frankincense, but answers can be sought in any type of incense.

My preferred method is a direct scrying technique based on looking for patterns and images in the smoke, rather like reading tea leaves. This method is discussed in more detail following the recipe for Ooky Spooky Evocation Smoke (see page 192). However, for people who prefer a more formulaic approach, I present this one modeled on the translation by Irving Finkel of the British Museum of an ancient Babylonian text. It provides sixteen specific omen interpretations. The tablet is badly damaged; there were probably originally thirty-two.

1. If when you sprinkle the incense its flame burns smokily, your army will defeat an enemy.

2. If when you sprinkle the incense it stops short, and afterwards its flame burns smokily, an enemy will defeat your army.

3. If . . . goes to its right and not to its left, you will prevail over your adversary.

4. If . . . goes to its left and not to its right, your adversary will prevail over you.

5. If . . . goes to the east and does not go towards the crotch of the diviner, downfall for your adversary.

6. If . . . towards the crotch of the diviner and not to the east, your adversary will prevail over you.

7. If . . . equally in all directions, equal weapons.

8. If . . . clusters: success: the man will enjoy profit wherever he goes.

9. If . . . fragmented, there will be financial loss and loss of livestock.

10. If the top of the incense is cleft: madness.

11. If the top of the incense is cut off, the man will experience hard times.

12. If the top of the incense looks like the brick-basket of Šamaš, there will be fever disease in the man's household.

13. If the top of the incense gathers like a date palm and is thin below, hardship will seize the man.

14. If the incense after a while is constricted, hard times will befall the man.

15. If the incense after a while pushes through and gets out, the man will pull through hard times.

16. If the incense pushes through to the east and gets out, the man will pull through hard times.

PSYCHIC SENSE INCENSE

This very simple incense is designed to facilitate astral vision, hearing, and other senses. This is a very light trance aid, which also makes a pleasant temple incense or offering to Asteria, the Titaness mother of Hekate and goddess of "night prophecy," including both astrology and oneiromancy.

2 parts frankincense to purify and clarify

3 parts jasmine to gently open the third eye

1 part dittany of Crete to aid vision across timelines

Honey to bind

TRANCE & JOURNEY AID

This is the incense I most often use when I want to open my senses for divination. It is a powerful aid to trance—too powerful for some people. If you find it easy to slip into trance but difficult to ground yourself when you're done, this is *not* the incense for you. If you, like me, are a bit of a control freak who has trouble letting go, then this can help ease the transition. It should be used only when you have time to devote to magic and you're in a safe place. Never drive or operate heavy machinery while you still feel the effects of this incense. For a stronger impact, you can lean into the smoke and huff it. If you do not have a trance practice already, my recommendation for the easiest trance state to learn is the one I call "Make Believe" or "childlike wonder." Breathe in the smoke, allow your imagination to come out, and give yourself permission to play. Don't try to force magic this first time. Just let your mind settle, open, and be. You may find it helpful to rock back and forth or spin around in circles until you are dizzy.

> 2 parts frankincense or another resin for enlightenment
>
> 3 parts mugwort to open the gates of trance
>
> 1 part amanita to expand consciousness
>
> 1 part clover flowers to open the road to the Other Place
>
> 1 part marijuana to elevate (optional)

PYTHIA'S ORACLE SMOKE

Pythia, of course, is not a proper name, but rather a title that was held by a number of women who served as oracle at Delphi in life. Πυθώ (Pytho) is the ancient name for Delphi, most likely derived from the Greek πύθειν (*pythein*), which means "to rot" or "to smell rotten." In ancient days, a foul-smelling vapor arose from the earth at Delphi, explained legendarily as the stench of the great dragon/serpent rotting below, who was named Πύθων (Python, the root of our English word). This vapor was said by some to be the foundation of the priestess's oracular trance. Likely because the underground aquifer has been diverted by human construction, the vapor no longer arises. Pythia, as I work with her, is not a single human, but rather an egregore spirit participated in by all those who became Pythia while they lived, giving up their name and their family and their essential individuality, to get slowly infused with the essence of Pythia, who lives forever in the Underworld. The vapors of Pytho were poison; they carried up the Python Voice, but each time they were breathed, they carried a tiny piece of the priestess down to live among the dead. It was a dangerous vocation.

A Nontoxic Incense to Help Hear and Speak with the Pythian Voice

> 3 parts resin (Myrrh is especially nice.)
>
> 2 parts mugwort or another artemisia
>
> 1 part bay (If you can get bay leaves from Delphi, add one.)
>
> 1 part dittany of Crete
>
> 1 tbsp marijuana flowers per ½ cup incense (optional, if legal, etc., etc.)

TAROT CONSECRATION SMOKE

This formula is designed to cleanse, bless, and empower tarot cards, runes, and other divination tools. For most tools, you can pass them through the smoke, but if you're concerned that it will damage them, then you can instead bury the tool in unlit incense. I do this for new tools, and otherwise only occasionally, when they feel sticky, dirty, or when they are not reading well. While this is a pleasant incense to burn while reading, I prefer Oracle Smoke for that.

> 3 parts mixed resins to lend the Sun's illuminating perspicacity
>
> 2 parts night-blooming jasmine to lend the Moon's intuitive premonition
>
> 3 parts star anise to lend the enlightening rays of the stars
>
> 1 part citrus peel for clarity
>
> 1 part thyme for the courage to speak the truth
>
> Honey to bind (This incense wants a lot of smoke, so the only limit to how much honey you add is that it not be too sticky to handle.)

Consecration Ritual for a New Deck

Some people believe that you should never buy a tarot deck yourself. Others believe that you should never use a tarot deck that has been handled by anyone but you. We all have our own particular superstitions, but broadly there are no universal rules about how to work with divinatory tools. For me, personally, I don't usually cleanse my cards unless I sense they are feeling energetically sticky and the same handful of cards show up over and over in different readings. I also cleanse used decks only if I don't like the way they feel from their old owner. Many people recommend cleansing your cards as soon as you get them and every full moon thereafter. Certainly, that seems like a very sensible strategy as well. As you work with your tools, you'll find your own rhythm together. In the ritual below, I'm blessing tarot cards, but this is easy to modify and equally effective with almost any kind of divinatory tool.

Begin by lighting the incense. As the smoke builds, handle your cards. Fan them out. Thank them for all they've done for you in the past.

Speak some kind of words to the Fates or whatever powers aid your divination. Speak from your heart, or choose a poem or prayer that feels right for those powers. Below is my translation of the Orphic hymn to the Fates, which you may use, with or without your own modifications. If you use it, try to follow the location of the poem in your imagination. Flow with the waters of Fate's deep well, down, down, down, into the Earth. Bubble up as a spring and fly out over the face of the Earth, and back down the ancestors.

Endless infinity, children of inky Night,

Fates, Providence, Moirai, I call you to this rite!

O many-named ones of the heavenly pools,

Whose warm waters burst forth like shining white jewels,

Everflowing by night, into the grotto,

In the whole holy hole's innermost hollow.

You first bubble forth from spiritual places,

From whence you fly forth o'er earth's boundless spaces,

then, nimble and quick, you scamper on down,

To be with the Ancestors, under the ground.

O Atropos, Who Must Be!

O Lachesis, Assigner of our destiny!

O Klotho, who Weaves all that we see!

Nocturnal, eternal, invisible, implacable,

You are indestructible and all-unattackable.

All things you give, and all things you stay,

And you are they who take all things away.

You who are the contingent and the necessary things:

Fates, hear my prayers, and hallow my offerings!

As these cards pass through the hallowing smoke,

I ask you to embrace them inside your cloak,

Hold them close to your heart and bless them with your grace,

That I may use them to speak Truth in the name of the Fates.

OOKY SPOOKY EVOCATION SMOKE

This smoke is designed to provide a heavy medium for spirits to manifest within. It is excellent for dark-mirror conjurations, one method for which I will teach below. You can customize this recipe for individual spirits by applying the techniques you learned in the Offerings for Named Spirits section. If you are especially trance-prone, this incense might be too much for you. Leave out the marijuana and replace half the wormwood with mugwort.

3 parts wormwood for spirit conjuration

2 parts resin to keep things from going too dark and provide a higher
     vibration (For necromancy, use myrrh. For angels use frankincense.)

1 part star anise to open the psychic senses and lend some clarity

1 part dittany of Crete to facilitate communication across timelines

½ part marijuana (optional)

Grind the ingredients together to a fine powder, and split this into thirds. Mix two-thirds of the powder with honey until a thick paste is formed. Roll into small balls; make a variety of sizes for different uses. Roll the balls in the remaining powder until they are no longer sticky. If the honey and resin are omitted, this recipe, boiled in spring water, forms an excellent basis for a fluid condenser.

Dark-Mirror Conjuration

YOU WILL NEED

> A large mirror, preferably pre-enchanted
>
> A black permanent magic marker
>
> A large clear table
>
> Two candles
>
> Incense (Ideally the incense above, but anything that produces a lot of smoke and is relevant to the work at hand will work.)
>
> About an hour of uninterrupted time (Mondays, Saturdays, and dark moons are good times for this work, particularly when you're first learning.)
>
> A seemingly random source of white noise that changes over time, such as rain or wind or ocean waves (It is okay to use a synthetic noise, but it has to be something that changes randomly over time. Prerecorded sound won't work.)
>
> Windex and rags

WHAT TO DO

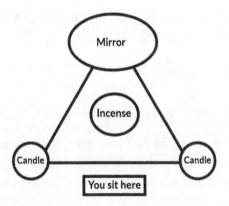

Arrange your workspace in an equilateral triangle, so that you can sit with one side right in front of you. At the far point of the triangle, prop up your mirror so that you can see yourself in it. At the center of the triangle, put the incense. The goal is to look through the cloud of incense into the mirror. Put the candles at the remaining two corners, so they flicker in your peripheral vision when looking into the mirror.

Choose a spirit with whom you would like to make contact through the mirror. When you're first learning, it's wise to start with a spirit you're reasonably confident likes you. I would recommend against the recently dead until you have more practice; those connections can be emotional and difficult to control. Hermes Philanthropos, Hermes the Friend of Humans, is a nice choice. He likes pretty much everyone, and he's chatty. Find or write an invocation for that spirit. For Hermes, I'd recommend his Orphic hymn, which is number 28. Prepare an offering. Minimally this should include cool, clean water and something nice to eat.

Just before beginning, draw a seal or symbol relevant to the spirit on the mirror. Draw it big, so it covers your face when you look in the mirror. For example, if you're calling Hermes, you could use ⚕, the caduceus. Light the incense and the candles. You'll want more incense handy, as you'll need to feed it as the rite progresses.

- Begin by entering magical space, time, and consciousness by any method.

- Close your eyes.

- Chant the invocation several times, entering deeper and deeper into trance. Rocking back and forth can help.

- With your eyes already closed, imagine closing a second, inner set of eyelids.

- Call, asking the spirit to appear in the mirror and to speak truly to you.

- Open your inner eyelids, and then your outer ones. Try to keep your eyes unfocused and look through the smoke into the mirror. If you're having trouble, rapidly switch focus from the incense cloud to the symbol to your eyes reflected in the mirror. Try to focus on all three of them at once, until you're focusing on none of them at all.

- Introduce yourself and explain why you have called. "To speak with you and seek your wisdom" is a good all-purpose reason, but it's better if you can be more specific.

- Ask the spirit if it is present. Watch the cloud of incense spiral and spin. Listen to the rain pitter-patter. Watch for the face as the incense smoke gyres and gymbles in the wabe. Listen for the voice in the rain. Be patient. Learning to see and hear in this way takes time. Don't speak. Just listen.

- Once you sense a response, begin to ask questions. As before, wait patiently for a response. It will get easier to sense with practice.

- Be sure to ask, before the conversation ends, if there is anything you can do for them. Say thank you, and then make your goodbyes.

- After the call ends, use Windex and a rag to wash away the symbol. If necessary, you can do this prematurely to end a call, but hanging up is rude and it's better to avoid it if possible.

- Remember to drink some water when you're done. This is thirsty work.

- Take some time to write some notes, and then eat something to help you ground.

- After that, do something entirely mundane, but that requires careful attention, like bookkeeping. If you let your mind wander too much, the work won't properly seal. The bookkeeping will prevent that. Be careful to record any dreams the night after a conjuration.

Cleansing & Protection

Throughout this section, we'll learn several types of cleansing and protection magic. However, before we get to that, I'd like to talk a little bit about why I'm reluctant to even teach this material. In my experience, almost all witches banish too much and employ too much protection. We all live in a dumpster-fire culture of rampant cursing. I can almost guarantee that you've been cursed at least once this week. For most people with healthy spiritual psyches, most of those curses are just background noise. In just the same way, every breath of air you take is swarming with germs, but most of them aren't a problem.

Many people wrap themselves in layers and layers of magical protection, even in the absence of any kind of specific threat. In my circle, we call that "wearing plate mail to a picnic," and all it does is make you look like easy prey or like a lunkhead spoiling for a fight. People who are confident in their own personal power do not need to go around draped in protection. Just as the best protection from disease is an intact skin and a healthy immune system, the best magic protection is to address your psychic trauma and live in right relationship with the world around you.

Of course, there are times when more aggressive protections are called for. When in dangerous circumstances, your best bet is a single simple layer of protection—metaphorically, a mask—and regular prophylactic cleansing—metaphorically, washing your hands. I recommend regular salt baths—once a month for most people or once a week for people in the public eye. Every day would be only for people who attract a lot of negative attention. The *most* important kind of magical protection is simply to keep your wits about you and be prepared to react when something actually does happen. When something weird happens, don't be complacent, but also don't freak out.

AGAINST FEAR

This recipe was given to me by Artemis, specifically to ward off fear. It is an excellent choice before going into battle—whether literal or metaphorical—and immediately afterward to aid trauma healing and reintegration. It is also useful to soothe fears that creep up from nowhere or occasional nightmares. It is *not* appropriate as a long-term treatment for anxiety disorders or PTSD.

> 3 parts frankincense or any other resin for the light of the sun, to
> illuminate dark shadows, and to make bright the way
>
> 2 parts thyme for bravery and battle spirit
>
> 1 part rosemary for courage
>
> 1 part lemon balm to gladden the heart
>
> Honey to bind

This incense is an excellent accompaniment to the following spell, partially inspired by PGM VII 686-702. You will notice it is very similar, but not identical to, the spell presented with the Great Bear offering incense on page 180. That is intentional; I wanted to show you how the same original source can be adapted to multiple purposes. While it can be performed anytime, it is especially potent under a clear night sky, with Ursa Major visible in the sky.

Light the incense, and enter into magical space, time, and consciousness. Speak from your heart, saying something like:

> Bear, Great Bear, you who rule the heavens, the stars, and the whole world, you who make the axis turn, I call on you for protection. Look after me, as a mother bear for her cubs. Defend me, as a mother does her cubs. Protect me, Great Bear Mother. I call upon you by your holy names. Brimo, Earth-breaker, Huntress Queen, Baubo, Midwife, All-Queen, Wish Queen, Queen of Witches, Great Bear of the North, Man Conquering, She of Lake and Cave, Priestess of the First Throne, Kallisti, Artemis, Hekate, Iphigenia, Great Lady of Beasts: I call on you as a little bear cub. Protect me, Great Bear!

PLAGUE DOCTOR'S MASK

This incense is perfect for fumigating a sickroom or anywhere else that bad vapors have collected. It is based on traditional medieval recipes for herbal stuffing to go inside a plague doctor's beaked mask, intended to filter out disease. It is not intended to treat any particular illness, but rather to provide a clean, comforting scent to calm the mind and raise the spirits. As always, avoid burning incense around people with respiratory illness. All smoke, because it introduces small particulates into the air, is bad for your lungs. This blend can also be boiled in water to produce a scented steam or brewed as a tea—although you will probably want to adjust the proportions to your particular tastes for that and omit the cedarwood. It can also be used in a cloth bag in the bath.

3 parts citrus peel for refreshing, clearing, and cleaning

1 part juniper needles for the crisp clean of a winter wood

1 part cedarwood for comfort, homeyness, and warmth

1 part thyme for courage and healing

1 part rosemary for healing and comfort

1 part sage for healing and spiritual cleansing

REBALANCING TONIC

As I mentioned before, I firmly believe that cultivating a healthy, harmonious, flourishing spiritual ecosystem is more or less the same as cultivating a biological one, and routine banishing is not conducive to that. Instead, I like to simply encourage the sort of spirit environment I want around me. A home that is full of good spirits/vibes just doesn't have room for bad ones. When things feel a little out of whack, this incense, combined with mundane cleaning, will normally bring things back into balance.

> 2 parts resin (Nothing disinfects like sunshine, and resin is sunshine made solid.)
>
> 1 part thyme for courage, crispness, and its anti-pest properties
>
> 1 part cedar for anti-pest properties and as the cool clean of a rich, damp forest
>
> 1 part clove against the evil eye and to help circulate energy and keep a space from becoming stagnant
>
> 1 part bay for brightness, clarity, and good order

BROAD-SPECTRUM CLEANSE

Sometimes things start to go wrong all at once. At such times, the best thing to do is to start some first-aid clearing and then diagnose what's going on. For a first pass at cleaning, take a hot bath in salt water while burning this incense. You can also put some of the incense in a cloth bag and add it to your bath. Do not add it directly to the bath; it's difficult to clean.

> 1 part camphor
>
> 3 parts cedar
>
> 2 parts hyssop
>
> 2 parts rosemary
>
> 4 parts lemon peel

Once you're out of the bath, do a little divination to investigate. My favorite tarot reading for diagnosing crossed conditions is below. Begin by clearly describing, in writing, the symptoms and occurrences that make you suspect crossed conditions. Then, after your normal divination preparations, deal out three cards:

WHAT is going on? What is the true nature of the situation described?

WHY is it happening? Why have these events happened?
Why do I feel this way?

HOW can the situation be improved? How should I proceed?
How can I fix it?

In general, Minor Arcana cards, particularly in the first position, indicate that there is nothing supernatural afoot.

Depending on the results of the divination, you may want to employ more sophisticated magic.

I'M RUBBER, YOU'RE GLUE

I developed this blend to accompany my favorite reversing spell. It's among the first spells I ever learned. This is just a slightly souped-up version of the spell you too learned as a kid. Because it is bound with glue, the incense cannot be stored; it should be made up fresh before each use. For this reason, I made sure to use only ingredients you are likely to already have on hand, but you can substitute as needed. The ratios are very flexible and largely depend on the freshness and particularity of the ingredients. Grind everything very fine.

> 3 parts onion or garlic peels
>
> 1 part rosemary, sage, or another salvia
>
> 1 part mugwort, tarragon, or another artemisia
>
> 1 part cloves
>
> Nontoxic school glue or library paste to bind

I'm Rubber, You're Glue Reversing Spell

YOU WILL NEED

> A photo of your target
>
> The incense above or a similar blend and a way to burn it in a large bowl
>
> A glass of water

WHAT TO DO

- Baptize the picture as your target.

- Coat the picture in a thin layer of glue.

- Put the photo, glue side up, on the table in front of you.

- Put the incense between you and the photo, and light it.

- Chant: "I'm rubber, you're glue! Everything you send bounces off of me and sticks to you!" several times, with increasing power. Get mad. When you are ready . . .

- Pick up the photo and hold it above the smoke, bathing it in the smoke, until the glue is coated in soot.

- If you would like to address specifics, such as, "Every lie you spread about me will be known about you!" now is the time to do it.

- Keep chanting, forcefully.

- When you feel the power peak, drop the photo onto the charcoal and watch it burn.

- Pour the water over the top of this.

- Throw out the mess, take out the trash, and then carefully wash your hands.

CLOAK OF INVISIBILITY

This incense is designed to operate with the spell below, which is inspired by PGM I 222-231.

3 parts frankincense

2 parts mugwort

2 parts dittany of Crete

1 part juniper needles

1 part hyssop

Honey to bind

YOU WILL NEED

The above incense and a way to burn it

A flat representation of the thing you want to hide, such as documents, pictures, or written descriptions

A glass cake dome

A white, black, or gray scarf large enough to cover the dome

WHAT TO DO

◆ Enter into magical space, time, and consciousness by any method.

◆ Baptize the representation as the thing it represents. The more tightly you can link them, the better.

◆ Put the representation faceup on the table.

◆ Put the incense brazier over top of the representation.

◆ Light the incense; if the smoke wanes while you are still working, add more. This spell wants a lot of smoke.

◆ Recite the Orphic hymn to Helios (below) several times until you "catch the vibe."

◆ Move your hands through the smoke like a magician, while saying (something like):

Helios, All Seeing Eye, I call you by your great name, BORKE PHOIOUR IO ZIZIA APARXEOUCH THYTHE LAILAM AAAAAA IIIII OOOOO IEO IEO IEO IEO IEO IEO IECO NAUNAX AI AI AEO AEO EAO.

◆ With the incense still burning, put the dome over it.

◆ Put your hands on the dome, and say (something like):

Make _____ invisible, lord Helios, AEO OAE EIE EAO, unseen and unknown to every person. IO IO IO PHRIXRIZO EOA.

◆ Place the scarf over the dome.

- Say (something like):

  Come, Darkness, who appeared in the beginning, and hide what is to be hidden!!

- Exit magical space, time, and consciousness.

- Go take a shower.

The Orphic Hymn to Helios

Hear me, blessed one, eternal all-seeing eye,

Gold gleaming light, Titan Most High,

You are self-made and tireless, of beautiful form:

On the right side, you give birth to the morn,

While with your left hand you pour out the night,

Compounding the hours, endless alchemy of light.

Your four fleet-footed horses gambol and play,

High-spirited coursers leading light of new day.

Whizzing blissful and swiftly, fiery charioteer,

Whirl like a bullroarer on your endless road round the year!

Draw forth cosmic harmony, good guide of the good,

Scorch the wrongdoers, who act in falsehood.

You give the signal, and good deeds are done,

You measure the seasons with revolutions you run.

Multiformed and evergreen, eternally undefiled,

Lightbringer, life-giver, cosmocrat, all-fruitful Paian.

You are immortal Zeus, and undying Father Time,

Truth-doing, all-shining, round-running cosmic eye.

You measure seasons, making sense, giving signs,

When the sun sets, and when you rise up and shine.

Flow-loving cosmic king beaming righteous light,

Truth-guarding all-protector, radiant knight,

Whip-whistling horse rider, life-loving charioteer:

Attend to my prayer, and to your mystics, draw near.

GHOST BUSTER

The most common kind of haunting I see isn't really a haunting at all: it's a kind of infection. When we die, most of the time, our psychic bonds dissolve within the first year after death. However, that process can go wrong, especially when the bonds were unhealthy in life and the person has died a bad death. In those cases, sometimes a small piece of the dead person can break off and become lodged in a living person or a physical object or location. This is most common when the death is that of a family member or other loved one with whom you had a difficult or abusive relationship in life. Although often called a haunting, it's not exactly that. There is not enough of the dead person left to have much personality; their primary "feelings" are that they are hungry and cold. The infection isn't a person; it's a piece of a thing that used to be a person. If you have eyes to see, this often looks like physical wounds, frequently with some kind of shrapnel stuck in them. They may appear infected or oozing. The incense recipe below is a gentle healing and cleansing for this sort of infection. Relax, center yourself, inhale the incense, and as you breathe out, try to push the spirit out of you. Ideally, do this while you are sitting in a salt bath. If this sort of home remedy does not work, you will need to consult a specialist. Depossession is a complicated procedure I cannot teach you here.

Expect grief—often complicated grief—to follow such a depossession. This can be the case even when the haunting spirit was not known to you in life. It's natural to feel sadness, anger, guilt, relief, shame, hope, and/or fear after a depossession, sometimes all at the same time. Everyone experiences grief differently; don't beat yourself up for not "doing it right." Whatever you're feeling is what you're feeling; don't judge yourself for it. Just give yourself some time and space to feel it. Journaling or talking about your feelings with someone else can help. If the feelings persist longer than seems right to you, seek advice from an expert.

This incense can also be used as a suffumigation to clear a haunted room or item. Those types of hauntings are often impacted, and sometimes require more sophisticated interventions. However, this incense can still be a good stopgap measure to quiet the symptoms. You will need a lot of this incense; it's best to burn enough that there is a visible cloud of smoke. For an infected place, close the doors and windows and hot box it until there is so much smoke it becomes difficult to breathe, then extinguish the incense, leave, and let it settle for a while. When the smoke clears, wash everything down with salt water.

> 2 parts frankincense
>
> 2 parts tarragon
>
> 1 part clove
>
> 1 part garlic or onion peels

If you like, accompany the fumigation with the recitation of an appropriate hymn. The Orphic hymn to the Titans (below) is my go-to, but Psalm 91 would also be nice.

Titans! Splendid children of Earth and Sky,

Eldermost ancestors, in Earth's womb you lie.

From the innermost nooks of the Great Below,

Timeless and ancient, you eternally flow.

Asleep deep beneath Tartarean soil,

You gave birth to all mortals who suffer and toil:

The maritime, the feathered, those of the earth,

Every life in the cosmos, you brought to birth.

I summon you now, and I beg you approach:

grant a divorce from all difficult ghosts.

BATTLEFIELD PROTECTION WITH
THE ANGELS OF THE SECOND HEAVEN

This incense is developed from *Sepher h'Razim* (Book of Secrets), a goetic Jewish grimoire from late antiquity. Legendarily, this book was given to Noah by the angel Raziel, whose name means "Secret of El." Long lost, the book was rediscovered by modern scholars by piecing together fragments found in genizoth, Jewish book coffins. The book is divided into seven sections, each of which lists the angels of one of the seven heavens. This spell is in the ninth step of the Seventh Heaven and produces a phylactery to provide protection in battle. This can be understood both literally and metaphorically. These are the phylacteries I make for protesters.

RECIPE

> 3 parts frankincense or other resin
>
> 2 parts bay
>
> 1 part spikenard or another valerian

YOU WILL NEED

> Incense and a way to burn it
>
> A scroll case
>
> A small strip of paper that, when rolled, will fit in the case
>
> A pen (If you have a magical pen, use that.)
>
> Plastic cling wrap
>
> A large scarf, such as a tallis or pashmina
>
> About an hour on a Tuesday while the sun shines

WHAT TO DO

♦ Arrange yourself with the scarf over your head in such a way that it narrows your vision to the cloud of incense. Enter into magical space, time, and consciousness. Light the incense. Stare into the glowing charcoal from a safe distance. Say the following or something like it out loud, while you write it on one side of the scroll:

Angels of the second heaven, you who stand upon the ninth step, I, NAME, child of NAME, SOME FANCY TITLES, call out to you. You quick and mighty ones, flying through the air! I, NAME, child of NAME, call to you. Your strength is a breastplate and you have swords in hand, grasping bows and holding javelins. Prepared for war, you leap from the flame on horses of flame, with harnesses of flame on chariots of fire. Terror goes with you, wherever you go. Let the phylactery protect from bullet and tear gas, arrow, sword, and any blow. Let it protect the entire body, mind, and spirit of NAME, child of NAME, now and forever more.

◆ Turn the phylactery over and say the names of the angels, while writing them on the reverse side of the scroll.

לאידודג	Gedvedial
לאיסכס	Saxial
לאינוסרת	Thrasuniel
לאיתצנ	Natziel
אדצא	Asdah
אינבר	Rabbiniah
לאלילה	Halilal
לאיפקות	Thackfiel
לאיכמס	Samkiel
לאהדפ	Padhal
אברק	Qarba
לאיצ	Ziel
לארפ	Pirel
לאיהתפ	Fethial

◆ Turn the scroll over, and read the first side again.

◆ Turn the scroll over, and read the angel names again.

◆ Turn the scroll over, and read the petition a third time.

- Turn the scroll over, and read the angel names a third time.

- Hold the scroll in both hands over the incense, and speak from your heart, praying with the angels of the ninth step of the Seventh Heaven. You may find yourself moved to sing or hum. That's a good impulse; go with it.

- When you feel the energy crescendo and abate, say thank you, and wish the angels goodbye.

Carefully wrap the scroll in the plastic cling wrap, overlapping the edges on the side with the petition. This will protect your scroll from rain and quick dunkings. If you're lucky, it will protect it from a spin cycle as well, but try not to test your luck. Roll the scroll up with לאידודג on the outside. Make sure the roll is tight enough to fit in the case.

Have the protectee wear it on their person, ideally on a string around their neck or in a breast pocket, so that it is near to their heart. I like to use a red string for extra luck and protection.

Glamour, Love & Emotional Healing

The incenses in this section are designed to help restore love and to attract potential partners. To force feelings in another person, you can try some of the options in the malefica section, but I generally recommend against it. The honey pot spell is excellent combined with almost all of those spells; you can add any of these incenses directly to the honey.

SUNSHINE HAPPINESS JOY BRINGER

This is one of my favorite blends. It's designed to infuse healing joy directly into the person smelling it. It is particularly nice while in a bath following difficult or emotional work. It can also be used to help send joy to someone else. This incense is a good choice when old ladies like me find that the "cold has gotten into our bones." This mixture is also nice as an offering to solar spirits. This incense is not a treatment for serious depression—although it might help a little!

3 parts mixed resins (I especially like Chios mastic in this for a sort of
   Greek island feel.)

2 parts citrus peel (A mixture of several types is nice.)

1 part dried coconut to make this incense smell like a tropical paradise, or
   at least like fancy sunscreen

1 part jasmine flower for the breath of a luxurious summer night

1 part cinnamon (This mix really rewards the use of high-quality Ceylon
   cinnamon, but grocery store cinnamon is also fine.)

This incense, which is very loosely inspired by one from *Sepher h'Razim*, is excellent combined with the following spell, best begun about half an hour before sunrise on a Sunday morning. It is designed to be cast for oneself, but could be adapted to use a poppet to cast on someone else.

Before beginning, bathe and dress in something festive. Arrange the incense above, a candle (preferably beeswax), a bell (preferably brass), and a knife (preferably obsidian) in a pleasing way so that you can reach them while standing (ideally outside, facing east).

Light the candle and incense. Enter into magical space, time, and consciousness. Hold your hands up and say this or something like it:

I, NAME, child of NAME, cry out to the angels of the fourth firmament, that castle upon the storm clouds, founded on pillars of fire, crowned with diadems of flame, full of treasures of strength and storehouses of dew. Prancers, dancers, wild ones, innumerable angels of the seven rivers of fire and water, I, NAME, call out to you now. Come and chant with me! Glory in the Life of the World!

Repeat the following list of names until the sun begins to rise:

Persial, who leads the sun by night, I, NAME, call you.

Abrasax, who leads the sun by day, I, NAME, call you.

Libbial, angel of the heart, I, NAME, call you.

Tzedekiel, angel of compassion, I, NAME, call you.

Nevimiel, angel of prophecy, I, NAME, call you.

Every angel of the fourth firmament, I, NAME, call on you in the name Shaddai El Chai.

Once the first glimmer of sunset begins, say this or something like it:

Angels that lead the sun in the power of your strength on the heavenly paths to illuminate the world, by the One whose voice shakes the earth, who moves mountains in anger, who calms the sea with power, who shakes the pillars of the world with a glance, who sustains everything with an arm, who is hidden from the eyes of all the living, who sits upon the throne of greatness of the kingdom of the glory of holiness, and who moves through the entire worlds, I call by the great, fearful, powerful, majestic, forceful, mighty, holy, strong, wondrous, secret, exalted, and glorious names that you will do my will and desire at this time and season and reveal to me the healing glory of the sun, without terror or injury.

Bask in the rising sun, feeling its power awaken you once more to joy. If you wish, you can make specific requests of the sun at this time by saying this or something like it:

Holy Helios who rises in the east, good mariner, trustworthy leader of the sun's rays, reliable witness, who of old established the mighty wheel of the heavens, holy orderer, ruler of the axis of heaven. Lord, Brilliant Leader, King, Soldier. I, NAME, child of NAME, present my supplication before you: MAKE YOUR REQUEST HERE.

When you are done communing with the sun, say thank you and this or something like it:

Blessed Angels, I call you in the name of the ONE who formed you in splendor and glory to illuminate the worlds that you will not harm me, and will not terrify me, but that we always be bound together in love and healing. I shall neither fear nor tremble nor cry, for you are with me.

Amen and Selah.

HEART HEALER

Brokenheartedness is a very real thing. It can be caused not only by the end of a love affair, but also by the loss of a family member or friend or even a more abstract situation, like the loss of self-identity that comes with losing a job. A broken heart is an actual, palpable wound to your psychic body, and it needs time and care to heal properly. If you try to ignore the wound or don't care for it properly, it can fester, ultimately poisoning you from within. We all know someone who's become so infected by the bitterness and bile from their broken heart that it slowly infected their whole soul. And yet, we also know, deep inside ourselves, that broken hearts can and do heal, leaving us strong and whole again. Sometimes, this process requires only time and rest. The body has a remarkable ability to heal itself with little intervention on our part. And yet, many injuries cannot heal themselves, and so we have invented medicine. Similarly, for psychic wounds, we have a remarkable ability to heal ourselves. And yet, it's not always enough. And so, we invented magic.

Shortly after my parents died, I was doing some meditations where the energy body is understood as a landscape that can be traveled through. For example, the cauldron of the womb—sometimes called the sacral chakra or the *dan tien*—I usually imagine as an opalescent sea that smells like tangerines and feels just like a hot tub with bubble jets. Similarly, I've always imagined the heart chakra to be a lush summer forest. That time, while I meditated, I began to feel the forest being cut down. I heard the chain saws and smelled smoke. I couldn't stop it, and soon the forest of my heart was leveled. And that's when I understood that a broken heart isn't a metaphor. My heart had been damaged and required mending. This incense is one of the many pieces of magic that helped me through.

4 parts frankincense for sunny lightness and gloom-lifting powers

2 parts rose petals for their association with love and their gentle healing

2 parts hyssop for gentle healing

1 part citrus peel to cut through the fog

1 part rosemary for remembrance of good times

1 part hawthorn to heal the heart

LOVE SPELL

This incense can be used in many ways. First, it is an excellent offering to any spirit of the sphere of Venus or anyone associated with romance and sex. It can be used as the basis of a variety of love spells, one example of which is presented below. It is delicious and delightful as a room scent, especially in the boudoir. It can also be ground fine and sparingly added to a honey cake for your beloved.

  1 part Chios mastic for the luxury of white sand and scintillating
    aquamarine water, for the sea-foam of Aphrodite's blest birth
  3 parts rose petals as love's own bloom, Queen of Flowers, the decadent
    and intoxicating smell of love
  2 parts apple blossom for the lightness and joy of initial infatuation
  1 part catnip to draw them in like catnip
  1 part damiana to ease anxiety, promote confidence, and set the mood
    for love
  1 part cinnamon for warmth to melt a frozen heart, and for a growing
    heat in the loins

PERFECT PARTNER DRAWING SPELL

Before performing the spell, spend some time really thinking about what you want in a lover. Make sure to include logistical necessities as this *really* is one of those "be careful what you wish for" deals. I've had these spells work perfectly, bringing me exactly what I asked for, except that I forgot to include something really important on the list . . . so he was married, or lived three thousand miles away, or was too young, or etc. Think it through, and write out your list. It's okay to be extremely specific, and don't be embarrassed to include shallower things or even things you think you're not supposed to want. It's even okay to put things down that seem to be in conflict with each other. The more specific, the better. Then, set your list aside for a day or two, and read it over again. Make sure it really is what you want.

YOU WILL NEED

Love Spell incense and a way to burn it

Your list

A seven-day novena candle in glass (Pink and/or rose-scented is best, but a plain white candle is fine. Virgin of Guadalupe candles are often pink and rose-scented and can be found in any grocery store in a Hispanic neighborhood. For this, however, peel the label off; you'll need to write on the candle jar. If it makes you feel weird to pull the label off, buy two, and burn the other for Holy Mother while explaining to her you needed the candle, but didn't mean to desecrate her image.)

A black permanent marker

About an hour of suspended disbelief, ideally on a Friday night while the moon waxes

WHAT TO DO

◆ Enter into magical time, space, and consciousness by any method.

◆ Using the marker, carefully write your list on the candle jar. Be sure to eyeball the length of your list and choose an appropriate size of writing to make sure it will all fit. If you have extra room, draw some hearts, seven-pointed stars, Cupid's arrows, Venus mirrors, or other love spell–looking symbols.

◆ Light the incense and the candle.

◆ Read the Orphic hymn to Aphrodite to the candle—not *at* the candle, *to* the candle. Treat the candle as if it has a real spirit in it, a personality all its own, one that loves and cares for you, and wants nothing more than to find you a great match.

◆ To level up this spell, you can dedicate the candle to a god or other spirit that rules over love. Promise them more candles and maybe roses, when the spell delivers. Make good on your promise when you get what you want.

◆ Read the hymn aloud again each night until the candle is gone.

♦ In my experience, it often takes another week or two after the candle is done for the right person to show up, but it's never been more than a month for me. Obviously, if you never leave your house, it will take longer. Go to a party, political protest, Gnostic Mass, museum gala, or somewhere else the sort of person you want to meet is likely to be.

♦ The goal of this spell is to meet a great partner. Actually courting them is up to you. I strongly discourage courtship magic. Every single time I've done it, I regretted it. Even when it works well, you'll always wonder: "Did I make them love me? Is this even real?"

JEZEBEL'S RED DRESS

This incense was designed for women who want to attract men and be seen as sexually desirable, but I have every reason to believe it will work for anyone regardless of gender or preference. The spell doesn't discriminate or vet what it attracts; it just turns up the sex. While I have never had this problem, others far prettier than I have reported that it draws unpleasant levels of attention and catcalling. Deploy with care.

Legendarily, Jezebel (לְבָזִיא), a princess of Tyre and queen of Israel by marriage, was a priestess of Baal and Asherah and instituted their worship in Israel. Her name derives from the holy cry לַעֵב וֹזִיָא (Ezo Baal)—which I have translated in the spell below as "Where is the Prince?"—which figures in ancient Semitic ritual practice similarly to how "weeping for Adonis" does in Greek and Roman paradigms. If you are not familiar with that mythology, you can think of it as similar to "John Barleycorn is dead!" in modern British paganism.

The first time I worked with Jezebel, I was getting ready to go out, and a little voice in the back of my head said, "No! Wear the red dress." It was a very successful outing. This incense can be ground fine and steeped to make a perfume oil or carried in the left pocket as a drawing talisman. Wearing a red dress is not strictly necessary to the operation of this spell; wear whatever you feel sexiest in.

1 part Chios mastic

2 parts sandalwood

3 parts rose

2 parts jasmine

1 part dried berries

1 part ginger

Jezebel Drawing Spell

Write a brief petition, outlining what you want. Light a red candle and the incense. Lie on top of the petition. Get in touch with yourself, if you know what I mean. As you feel the power build, just before climax, say this or something similar:

Jezebel, priestess of Asherah, priestess of Baal,

With you I cry out: Where, oh where, is the Prince?

Jezebel, Phoenician Queen, daughter of Ithobaal,

From the depths of Hell, rise up, rise up,

Jezebel, be with me tonight!

Where, oh where, is the Prince?

IN THE MOOD

This is a lovely, very sweet, and sensual blend. It can be used to set a mood in the bedroom or as an offering to spirits of the sphere of Venus, but it particularly shines in lust and desire spells. Its ingredients echo some used in Hoodoo blends like Kiss Me Quick! or Come to Me! and for the most part it can be used interchangeably with those blends for spellwork. It can be ground fine and added to sweet almond carrier oil to anoint candles. It is especially nice for this work to use candles shaped like genitals, which are readily available online or in any witch store. For a little kick, you can add one-half part cinnamon. For a bit more of a slow burn, replace half the damiana with tobacco.

3 parts damiana to increase desire and decrease inhibitions

1 part sandalwood for luxury and sensual delight

1 part jasmine for lust

1 part rose for love

1 part resin for joy

1 part dyktima for adventure

1 part dates for sweetness

Luck & Success Magic

FORTUNE'S FAVOR

This incense, which simply grants good luck, is applicable to almost any situation. After all, when don't you want better luck? It is quite similar to most blends called "fast luck" and can be used more or less interchangeably with them. This recipe, in particular, is designed to work with the help of the Greek goddess Tykhe (Τύχη), but could easily be adapted to function without her. Tykhe's name is usually translated as "Fortune," following her Latin name of Fortuna. The word τύχη itself comes from τυχανο, which means "to hit" in the sense of "to hit upon by chance," "to hit the jackpot," or "to hit a target."

In Greece, Tykhe had three main types of iconography, whom I generally think of as sisters. The joyful form called Eutykhia (good fortune) was often depicted holding a cornucopia and the babe Ploutos, the god of wealth. In her primordial form, Tykhe is often depicted with a ball of string, as one of the Moirae, the weavers of fate. Finally, in her dark form, Tykhe carries a sword and is called Nemesis (Νεμεσις). This word means "giver of fairness" or "reparation." She was the scourge of the wicked and the unjustly favored and checked her sister's extravagance to keep all in balance. That her name has come to mean "enemy" in English is the result of our culture's lust for unchecked greed and unfair accumulation of wealth and privilege. She is not the people's enemy.

4 parts frankincense or another resin

1 part mint—or wintergreen for a more "fast luck" feel

1 part cinnamon

1 part rose or another sweet flower

Luck-Bringing Spell

YOU WILL NEED

Pen and paper

10 coins (I like the gold-colored Sacagawea dollars for this, but any coins
will work. It is best not to be stingy, but if you are in hard times,
pennies are fine.)

A glass of water

A candle

Incense (The incense above is best, but plain frankincense is also okay.)

A tray or large plate on a table (A brass serving platter is perfect.)

About half an hour

As always, first decide exactly what you want. When you know exactly
what that is, write a letter to Tykhe requesting it. Write longwise along the
paper—this just makes the altar setup prettier, though; it's not essential.
Be as artful with the wording as you can, but do not trade off clarity for
poetics.

After you've written your petition, lay it down and arrange the ten
coins in a tetractys pyramid on top of it as follows: Use six coins to make
an equilateral triangle pointing at the ikon. Next, use three coins to make
another smaller triangle centered on top of the first one. Center the final
coin on top of that. On top of the central coin, place the incense charcoal—
unlit for now. To the side, put the water and candle. It's best to set all this
up in advance, and then enter magical space, time, and consciousness. Say
this or something like it:

> Tykhe, beautiful, powerful, and most-honored goddess, I have laid an
> offering of gold before you. I kindle flame for you. [Light the candle.]
> I burn sweet incense to you [light the incense], that its smell awakens
> and delights you. May these offerings be transformed into all those
> things you most desire! For these many fine offerings, I ask but a
> simple blessing, that DESCRIBE WHAT YOU WANT.

Sit in magical space, time, and consciousness, communing with Tykhe,
listening and feeling for a response. Watch the incense curl into faces. You
may also use any divination method you like to communicate with Tykhe

during this time. If you do not receive a clear response in the ritual, expect one in your dreams.

Keep a careful eye on the incense, so that you don't set the paper on fire. If it does start to burn? That's okay; that's why you have the glass of water. When you are done, pour the water over top and make sure everything is cold. This is why you need the tray, both to catch the water and to make sure you don't accidentally set the table on fire.

Over the next week, give away all ten coins, which carry a blessing of good luck, ideally to ten different beggars. If, at the end of the week, you still have coins left, you may leave those that remain at a crossroads or throw them into a wishing well or fountain, but putting them directly into the hands of less fortunate people while touching their hands, looking in their eyes, and conveying the blessing to them is better. When your request is fulfilled, you should give more in thanksgiving. Once granted, the petition may be ritually disposed of or kept in a petition box.

NIKE'S VICTORY WREATH INCENSE

Nike is the Greek goddess of victory. She is often pictured held in Zeus's hand. The most potent of Nike's symbols is the laurel wreath. The plant is closely associated with Apollo. At Delphi, it was chewed by the Pythian oracle while she prophesied. Additionally, it was awarded to the winners of both athletic and poetry competitions at the Pythian Games, a practice that has spread throughout our culture. To this day, the laurel wreath is so closely associated with victory that it is referenced in a number of English idioms. We say that someone is "resting on their laurels" when they are content to bask in previous successes and no longer have any ambition. We also use it in phrases for distinguished people such as "poet laureate" and "baccalaureate."

This incense is similar in both ingredients and use to Hoodoo blends often called "Crown of Success" and can be employed in almost any spell that calls for such.

3 parts frankincense

2 parts bay leaves (For extra potency, write Nike's name in Greek—

 NIKH—on the bay leaves before crushing.)

1 part cedarwood or another aromatic wood

Instead of preblending this incense, I also like to make an incense stack with the ingredients. Make a bed of gravel, dirt, sand, or salt. Cover it in some cedarwood chips, and lay the charcoal on top of that. Directly on top of the charcoal, put a bay leaf, with a sigil of your specific desire written on one side and Nike's name on the other. On top of the leaf, put a gold coin. On top of the coin, add some frankincense. After the incense is burned and the charcoal is cool, rinse off the coin and carry it as a victory charm.

CHARISMATIC AF

This incense is appropriate for all situations where you want to charm other people. It's excellent for use to psych yourself up before job interviews and first dates, as well as for any kind of performance. It is specifically designed to be used with the spell below, calling on the powers of the Graces (Χάριτες) to lend you their power for a specific time-bound endeavor like a performance or interview. It can also be used as an offering for the Graces.

> 3 parts resin to shine like the sun
>
> 2 parts rose so everyone loves you
>
> 1 part cloves so you're witty and clever and cool
>
> 1 part thyme so you're confident and courageous
>
> 1 part wildflowers for their simple charm (I like violets and clover, but whatever is local and fresh is good.)

And beautiful Eurynome [Wide Wandering], the daughter of Okeanos [Ocean], bore him [Zeus] three fair-cheeked Charities [Graces], Aglaea [Shining One], and Euphrosyne [Joy], and lovely Thalia [Bloom], from whose glancing eyes flowed love that unnerves the limbs; beautiful is their glance beneath their brows.

The Graces are goddesses of charm, charisma, and creativity. They are grace, personified. They grant the divine gifts we call charisma or poise. As in the quote above, from Hesiod's "Theogony," the Graces are generally understood as a trio of sisters, although their names and genealogies differ from storyteller to storyteller. In Greece, the Graces were called the Charites, a word closer in meaning to the English *charismatics* than to our word *charity*. They are very old goddesses, having been worshipped in the land we call Greece far before the Greek language arrived there. In this most archaic form, they are dancing nature spirits, especially associated with joy, fertility, and freshwater springs.

From ancient days up through the present, the Graces have a very consistent iconography. They are nearly always depicted as three beautiful young women dancing together, usually naked, but sometimes wearing filmy peploi, often with their arms draped across each other. This iconography is remarkably robust; whether painted by the ancients at Pompei or Sandro Botticelli or Pablo Picasso, whether classically sculpted in marble or cast in brutalist brass, the Graces are always recognizable. If you are not familiar with their iconography, look up several examples before you work the spell.

In this spell, we'll be employing a classic technique called "assumption of the god form" to borrow their charisma. Once you learn the technique, I think you will have no difficulty applying it to other gods and spirits with clear, well-established iconography. Assuming a god form is basically a way to realign your aura to be in harmony with a particular divine energy. It is an intermediary stage between imitation and channeling.

Think about what sort of grace you would like; perhaps make a list of qualities. For example, perhaps you want to be confident, witty, charming, intriguing, and unforgettable. Imagine what it would be like to have those gifts. Imagine people—real or fictional—that exemplify those characteristics. What about their behavior indicates they possess that particular grace?

Choose a famous representation of the Graces that most clearly speaks to you about the qualities you have chosen. Take some time to really study it, noting all the little details and understanding all the symbolism. If possible, visit your representation in a museum, but just looking at pictures online is good enough. There's no need to reinvent the wheel for this analysis; the reason I had you choose a famous representation was so that you could study what others have to say about it. When you feel as though you really know the piece, try to imagine inhabiting it. What does it feel like to be one of those Graces? Pick one in particular, and pose as her. Try to feel what it is like to be her.

Once you've done this studying and prep work, you're ready to begin the actual spell. Light the incense and a beeswax candle. Turn off all other lights. Enter into magical space, time, and consciousness. Make an invocation of the Graces, and explain why you are calling on them: to request a temporary infusion of charisma for your particular event. Close your eyes and imagine you are putting on your chosen Grace like a costume. Feel yourself slip into it. Dance with her sisters in her place. While you may choose to do this while sitting still, you may find it helpful to actually stand up and dance.

Once you feel that you are successfully wearing the Grace's skin, allow the essence to diffuse into your core. For the most part, this involves carefully centering and clarifying yourself, quieting your ego for a while to allow the god space to breathe. You may find yourself moved to dance again or to speak prophecy in the name of the Graces. Go with the flow.

Once you feel comfortable being the Grace, pour the feeling into a charm of some type. Jewelry is nice, but a special tie or even a lucky charm to keep in your pocket is good. It's also nice if the charm is thematically appropriate to the Graces, such as garlands, apples, roses, myrtle blossoms, or dice. It is relatively easy to find cameo jewelry depicting the Graces, if you think you'll be working with them often.

As the Grace, hold the charm in your hands, clasp it to your heart, breathe into it, and love it. Bless the charm with the gift you are request-ing. When you have exhausted all your power and cannot hold the form any longer, remember to say thank you and goodbye. Charms made in this way will not last terribly long. It's best to make them the day before you need them. More experienced magicians can easily adapt this technique for longer-lasting charms.

THREEFOLD WISHING

This spell can be adapted to almost all purposes. Unlike most incense blends in this book, this one is better unmixed. Add the incense ingredients in turn as the magic progresses. They will blend as they burn.

> Whole black peppercorns (Soak them in water for a while, so they burn slower. Three peppercorns is more than enough. *Never* burn ground pepper; that's basically just tear-gassing yourself.)
>
> White frankincense or another resin. (This spell will reward using the highest-quality resin you have.)
>
> Red rose petals

Before beginning, clearly articulate a three-point strategy for your wish.

What needs to be destroyed?

What needs to be created?

What do you want to grow?

For each question, it's okay to state something abstract, but the more specific and concrete you can be, the better. It's better if the three phases strategize together as well. For example: "destroy fat, create energy, grow muscle" or "destroy debt, create opportunity, grow wealth" or "destroy curses, create alliances, grow power." Form clear, simple, straightforward wishes for each phase before working the spell.

Devise or discover a small, easy-to-draw symbol or sigil to represent each of your three phases. Runes work well for this. Cut small circles of paper—I trace a quarter as a template—and put one sigil on each. Number them on the back, so you don't accidentally do them in the wrong order. Charge, but do not launch, the sigils.

This spell can be performed at any time but is particularly powerful during a lunar or solar eclipse. If working during an eclipse, time it so that the black phase occurs while it is getting dark, the white phase is during the total eclipse, and the red phase is while it is getting lighter. New moons or Saturdays are also good days for this work.

Arrange your altar with a flint knife, a small glass of whole milk, an egg, and one, three, seven, or thirteen red roses in a vase. Even better is a small potted rose you will tend. When you're ready, enter into magical space, time, and consciousness, and light the charcoal.

Say (something like):

Ἑκάτη Τριοδῖτις (Hekate Trioditus), Witch of the Threefold Way,

I call to you, Sorceress Queen, to work my will with me.

STATE INTENT HERE

Place the first sigil on the charcoal with the peppercorns. Say something like:

By blackest night, by flint-chipped blade, cut away that which
   fetters me.

Ritually cut a circle around yourself.

Do not continue until the first sigil is wholly consumed.

Place the second sigil and the frankincense on the charcoal. Say something like:

By white-shelled egg and creamy milk, bring forth that which I desire.

Take a sip of the milk, delighting in it, and then pour the rest over the egg.

Do not continue until the second sigil has been consumed.

Place the third sigil and the rose petals on the charcoal. If you wish, you may add a single drop of your own blood, but that is not required. Say something like:

By the reddest blood and rose's bloom, let my wish grow strong
    and true.

Do not continue until the third sigil has been consumed.

When all the sigils have fully burned, and you feel that you are done, say:

Torchbearer, Maiden, Goddess, Queen,

Guide me as I walk the threefold path.

Nigredo. Albano. Rubedo.

Goddess, Witch, Priestess.

While not strictly necessary, if you didn't work during an eclipse, I recommend repeating the spell three times. This can be on three consecutive days, once each week for three weeks, or on three consecutive new moons.

Money & Prosperity Magic

Money magic comes in five broad flavors, which I call Quick Cash, Money Healing, Debt Busting, Income Generating, and Wealth Building. They're each important, and long-term money work should involve all of them. If you find yourself constantly relying on Quick Cash magic, you should start working on the others to build a cushion. If you never find yourself in need of Quick Cash, you should probably be hoarding less and giving more away.

KA-CHING! QUICK CASH

Quick Cash work is for when you need a relatively small amount of money relatively quickly. What "relatively small" means varies from person to person, but we're mostly talking about an amount less than one month of your wages that you need in less than two weeks. This kind of magic is for when you just require a little bit extra to make ends meet. Be cautious: the money produced with this kind of magic can be very "easy come, easy go"; it is not a long-term solution. If you find yourself turning to this kind of magic month after month, you need to work in the other four categories as well.

Be sure to be alert for unusual opportunities when working this kind of magic; the money often appears in unexpected ways. For example, I once did some Quick Cash work with the Titaness Euphyressa, a Greek goddess of many powers; among them, it is she who "puts the glimmer in gold." The next day, I got an offer to write giantess erotica for cash. The gods work in mysterious ways, y'all!

> 2 parts frankincense to shine like the light of the sun on you
>
> 1 part tobacco, mostly as an offering to the luck spirits
>
> 1 part cinnamon to warm things up and get them flowing
>
> 1 part citrus peels to cut through the noise and make a path

$$¢¢$$ SPELL

In this spell, we'll be charging up a monetary bill to go out into the world as an ambassador on your behalf and recruit more money to come back to you. It is best cast in the hour of Jupiter on a Wednesday or an hour of Mercury on a Sunday, but it can be done anytime. This spell is inspired by one taught by Cat Yronwode on the Lucky Mojo Curio Company website.

YOU WILL NEED

Incense and a way to burn it

Two or more pieces of paper money (I like $2 bills—which you can get at
   any U.S. bank—but you can do it with any denomination of your own

local currency. If possible, choose a bill that is special or unusual in some way for at least one of them.)

A permanent magic marker (Metallic gold is best, but green or black is also fine.)

Soap and water

Begin by washing the bills carefully with soap and water. Allow them to dry in the sunshine. When you're ready, light the incense, and enter into magical space, time, and consciousness. Carefully, and with intention, write the success sigil, $$¢¢$$, diagonally in each corner of each bill, on both sides. Put your initials under the treasurer's signature. Hold the bills over the incense, and wave them back and forth in the smoke, praying for more money to come to you. Psalm 23 is a good choice, as is the Orphic hymn to Tykhe. However, in my opinion, it is always best to speak your own words directly from your heart, explaining your current hopes and fears. Keep praying and fumigating the bill until the incense goes out. It's just as easy to charge many bills as just two; there's no reason not to charge all the money you have on hand when you cast the spell. Tuck one bill carefully into your wallet, and spend the other(s) on something that will help you make money, such as office supplies or a work uniform. In my opinion, it is especially nice to spend it on gas or bus fare to get to work or an interview, because that helps open the roads to success for you.

MONEY HEALING

Our culture teaches us a lot of really gross and often contradictory stuff about money. You will *never* be in right relationship with money until you work through all of that. This incense is designed to be used with regular study, introspection, meditation, and shadow work to facilitate that healing. Caution: getting "woke" to how money works in our culture is not going to be fun, but it is necessary.

Frankincense to shine like the sun, exposing what has been hidden from you and disinfecting all corruption

Citrus peel to clarify and cut through all the grease and corruption.

Thyme to heal and offer the courage to look clearly at the realities of your situation

Wildflowers, especially clover (This is partly to remind you to find joy in this work, but also to remind you that the foundation of all wealth is land.)

MONEY MAGNET INCENSE

This incense can be used by anyone to attract more money, but it pairs best with non-magical activities that provide clear pathways for money to come in, such as a yard sale or side hustle or going to visit a rich uncle. It is best understood as advertising magic. Like most advertising magic, it draws on ingredients traditional to love magic to attract attention and inspire desire in combination with ingredients often used in magic related to wealth.

4 parts pine or another resin

2 parts cedar or another wood

2 parts rose

1 part cloves

1 part bay leaves

A Spell for Vending at Conventions or Other Events

This spell is designed to be done in the vendor's room after people have set up, but before the customers have arrived. Recruit as many other vendors as you can to work the spell together. You're not in competition with them; everyone does better when there are more people and when those people are in a buying mood. While designed to be performed by burning the incense above, it will also work if you sprinkle the loose incense around the space, which is often necessary because many venues do not permit incense. You will also need at least $8.88 in loose change, which you should scatter in the aisles.

Mercury, master of the marketplace,

Attend to our prayer and enter this space!

Celestial marketer, incline us your ear,

And rain down your luck on all gathered here.

We've shuffled our cards and laid out our wares,

Our cashboxes are open and so are our Squares.

For you do we offer this finest of incense,

and also eight hundred and eighty-eight cents.

God of merchants, magicians, diviners, and thieves,

Bring witches big riches beyond all our wishes,

Riches sufficient for a lifetime of ease.

A Khernips Spell for Getting Out of Debt

Khernips is a type of blessed holy water popular in Hellenic reconstructionist paganism. It is made by dropping burning herbs or incense into clean water and used to clean away the miasma of spiritual pollution. For this spell, you don't want to use charcoal, because it will pollute the water. I usually put the incense in a cast-iron pan lined with tinfoil and cook it on the stove until it starts to smoke. The formula below is my go-to for making khernips, but almost any incense will work. Grind everything very fine.

> 1 part pine or another resin
> 1 part bay leaves
> 1 part rosemary

YOU WILL NEED

> The incense and a clean way to burn it.
> 2 large glass or metal bowls or other deep containers (Bigger is better. At minimum, they need to be deep enough to completely submerge the poppet in.)
> Living water—that is, water collected from a natural source, like a river or rain
> An old towel you don't mind staining (This spell can be messy. It's easiest to do it outside.)

A small beeswax poppet of the person who is in debt, including as many
  links such as blood, hair, nails, photos, etc. as possible (If your poppet
  is not beeswax, that's okay, but it needs to float.)

A lead fishing weight on a short string

Documents relating to the debt like bills, etc. (These will be ruined; copies
  are fine.)

If possible, material links to your debt holders, such as a rock from the
  parking lot of your mortgage holder (Promotional materials with the
  bank, etc., logo on them are also good. Credit cards are also good.
  These are going to get stained.)

Six gold-colored coins (Sacagawea dollars are great. These coins will be
  blessed during the rite.)

Scissors

Red ink or paint

A handkerchief or other small cloth

PREPARATION

♦ Read this entire spell before you begin.

♦ Make a full accounting of all your debts. Write them down, and collect all the supporting data you can.

♦ Spend some time thinking about how you got into this situation.
   Did it happen slowly or quickly? Was it a medical crisis? Theft?
   Irresponsible spending? Write a letter to yourself, explaining what
   happened. Take responsibility and make a confession for the parts
   of it that are your fault, and make sure you've addressed anything
   that might happen again.

♦ Write a clear explanation of what you would like to have happen.
   What does salvation from your debt look like? Include a reasonable
   timeline. Rewrite it into a pretty petition.

♦ Arrange some towels under and around the container. This spell
   makes a mess.

- Prepare and baptize the poppet. Tie the weight to it with an inch or two of loose string between them.

- Prepare the "Red Ink of Debt":

    Line the bottom of your container with the debt documents and debt holder links, as well as your written letter to yourself.

    Fill the container halfway with water dyed red.

    Speak over the water, naming it Red Ink of Debt. Explain to it that it is the sea of debt in which you are drowning. Name all the debts. Explain how those debts have come to pass, and how they are damaging you, and what you need. Really feel it. If possible, cry into it. Spend some time on this step.

- Prepare the "Lustrous Water of Salvation":

    Line the bottom of the second container with your explanation of what you want and the six gold coins.

    Fill it with salt water.

    Speak over the water, naming it Lustrous Water of Salvation. Explain to it what its nature is. What does your situation look like after you are saved? Be specific, and use detail. Really feel it. If possible, cry into it.

- Arrange the petition, baths, incense, and poppet on your work surface.

THE RITUAL

- A Sun hour on a Saturday or Saturn hour on a Sunday are good choices for this work, but any time is okay.

- Enter magical time, space, and consciousness in the usual fashion.

- Light the incense.

- Drop the weighted poppet into the sea of debt.

- Yell at the Sea of Debt, speaking out loud your greatest fears and shame related to the debt. Really feel it. When you are crying out, at peak frenzy . . .

- Drop this incense into the Water of Salvation to activate it. Speak its name aloud once more: "You are the Lustrous Water of Salvation!"

- Cut the string, letting the poppet bob to the surface. Fish the poppet out, and wash it in the Lustrous Water of Salvation. While you wash it, say something like "You are rescued! Be pure of all debt!"

- Carefully, gently, and lovingly dry the poppet off and then wrap it in the handkerchief. Store it carefully for future use.

- The Lustrous Water of Salvation is best poured out at the base of a fruit tree or in a garden, but you may return it to the Land by any route, including by pouring it down a drain if necessary. Carefully dispose of the Sea of Debt. A toilet is a good choice, but you can also pour it onto the ground. Remember, it's full of ink, and not very good for plants. Pour extra water to wash it out.

- Exit ritual time, space, and consciousness as usual.

- Take all appropriate mundane actions to resolve your debt.

Autumn Wealth

Inspiration can come from strange places. This incense was inspired by the name of a fancy scented candle I saw advertised online. Struck by the name, I tried to imagine what Autumn Wealth might smell like, and I had an immediate sense of an incense as rich as a good harvest, golden with resin, highlighted by the luxury and wealth of the ancient Spice Road. Imagine my disappointment when, upon closer inspection, I found the candle was actually called Autumn Wreath, and I had simply misread it. In any case, the incense below truly is Autumn Wealth, and it's particularly good for spells to help you reap a good harvest, like the one below.

> 3 parts frankincense or another resin
> 1 part cinnamon

1 part cloves

1 part spicebush or allspice

1 part tobacco

A Spell to Reap a Good Harvest

Almost all agricultural magic can be adapted to any situation in which you've invested a great deal of effort in hopes that your investment will grow in value. When you are ready to harvest that effort, this spell can help. It's ideal for selling a house, but can also be used to get a promotion, a master's degree, or any type of capital gain. In the example below, I'll be using the spell to sell a house, but you'll see how to adapt it.

YOU WILL NEED

About an hour, ideally during the hour of Jupiter on a Saturday

A small glass of clean water

A bowl of dirt from a place relevant to the topic at hand

Incense and charcoal

A cookie, biscuit, or other small food offering

An initial offering of 9 identical coins, ideally "Three Sisters" coins

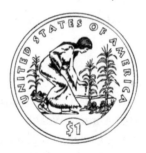

An additional offering for charity of $99 when the house sells. If you are adapting this spell for an alternate purpose, you can make an offering appropriate to the size of the request. If it's a cash offering, multiples of nine are a good choice.

Before beginning the spell, take some time to very carefully lay out exactly what you want to work for. Try to get your intent down to a single sentence.

In this example, I'll be doing "Sell this house for a profit." Use any method to develop a symbol or sigil to represent your goal. If you are using this spell to sell your primary residence, you can use the one below. Otherwise, you'll need to make your own. Trace a coin onto your paper and cut out a circle. Draw your sigil in the circle.

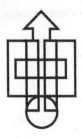

One top of the dirt, arrange six coins in a hexagon around the sigil, and then stack two coins on top of the sigil. Place the lit charcoal on top of the stack, and carefully place another coin on top of the charcoal. Sprinkle the incense liberally over this whole coin "flower."

Enter into magical space, time, and consciousness, and say something like:

> I present this golden flower as a symbol of my harvest. Faithfully have I maintained this property for NUMBER years, and improved it by LIST EXAMPLES. The time has come to harvest that value and move on. Dirt, gold, flower, flame, help me reap my harvest. Dirt, gold, flower, flame, help me reap my harvest . . .

Continue the chant until the incense is out—which is about thirty to sixty minutes for most types of charcoal. Make sure everything is cold before proceeding.

The top coin should be carried in your wallet until the goal has been accomplished. When your goal is achieved, throw it in a river, lake, fountain, or wishing well. The other eight coins may be either distributed to those in need or buried at the property in question.

WEALTH-DRAWING INCENSE

I'm kind of cheating a little bit with this recipe. While it can be burned as an incense, I more often use this blend as a potpourri. In particular, I sprinkle it in my cashbox when I vend and in an enchanted piggy bank, which I'll teach you how to make below.

3 parts juniper

2 parts dried figs or raisins

2 parts cedarwood or another aromatic wood

1 part roses

1 part whole black peppercorns

PLUTON & PERSEPHONE'S PIGGY BANK

We spoke before about the Queen of Hell's role as the overseer of the dead, but we touched less on her role as a wealth-bestower. All wealth arises from below, from the Land. Not just gold and gems, but also the bountiful fruits of the Earth; all wealth comes out of the ground. In the following work, which was loosely inspired by a 3rd-century Roman lead tablet, we call on Persephone under the name of her Sumerian counterpart Ereshkigal.

This spell is designed to slowly build prosperity over time. This is not a fast-acting spell, but a long-acting one; results will come with patience. Before beginning, light the incense and prepare yourself for magic in your usual fashion. If you have specific goals regarding prosperity, create a sigil—or a few sigils—to encode them.

Next, write the following on the other side of your sigil, while speaking the words aloud. It's okay to say the barbarous words however feels right to you, but try not to stumble over them. For this, it's better to be confidently wrong than timidly right.

Kore Ereshkigal, I invoke you by the name of the earth

KEUEMORI MORITHARCHOTH

Kore Ereshkigal ZABARBATHOUCH

Persephone ZAUDACHTHOUMAR

You who push seed to sprout, bud to flower, flower to fruit

You who are the Earth into which the fruit decays.

You who dwell beneath the Earth,

Ereshkigal NEBOUTOSOUALETH EREBENNE ARKUIA NEKUI

You who are bedecked with every jewel, crowned in gold and glory,

As ever your hoard of wealth grows, grow ever my prosperity as well,

For I am you, and you are me

I am Persephone, and Persephone is me.

I am the Queen who reigns in Hell, on Earth, in Heaven.

In all three worlds we are, she is, I am.

THREKISITHPHE AMRACHARARA EPHOISKERE

With this blood, I bind the spell.

Place a single drop of your blood on the paper to bind you to it and to seal the spell.

Put the paper, as well as a single gold coin, in the piggy bank. Sprinkle some incense on top as an offering. Each month, when the moon is full, open the box, light more incense, read the spell aloud again, and add another gold coin. Whenever you can, add more money to the piggy bank. The $$¢¢$$ dollars you enchanted in the earlier spell are a nice choice. You can also add things like banking or investment statements to the piggy bank, but *do not* add statements concerning debt.

Malefic Spells

Malefica, sometimes called black magic, is a broad category, and one with very fuzzy boundaries. For the most part, I consider all nonconsensual magic targeted at another person malefic. However, like all ethically sticky matters, things ought to be evaluated on a case by case basis. I most often use malefic in the context of political and social justice work.

NAIL IT DOWN!

This incense is designed to be used with the spell below to keep a piece of land from selling or from being developed. Historically, it is most often used by renters to prevent evictions and gentrification, but it can be applied in many other contexts as well, particularly as a form of environmental protest. For example, in my own practice, I use a slightly modified version of this spell at the local U.S. Steel mill, where they have been attempting to put in fracking wells for several years. The spell comes in two versions; one is designed for the short term—up to five years—while the other will prevent development "until iron rots." In general, I encourage you to use the long-term version only for natural land conservation. This spell is cast in three phases: making the incense, enchanting the spikes, and planting the spikes. These can be done in separate sessions or even by different people. Be sure to read this whole spell before starting.

Phase One: Make the Incense

> 2 parts resin (This should ideally be wildcrafted from the immediate vicinity of the land.)
>
> 1 part wood (This should ideally be wildcrafted from the immediate vicinity of the land.)
>
> 1 part artemisia for the spirits of the wild
>
> 1 part cloves because they look like nails and also add a spicy martial edge
>
> 1 sprinkle dirt from the grave of a righteous martyr (I use dirt from the grave of the workers killed in the Homestead Uprising, who were fighting Carnegie Steel—now U.S. Steel—when they were killed by union-busting mercenaries—now Securitas AB.)
>
> 1 sprinkle dirt from the grave of a robber baron (I use Andrew Carnegie's.)

The incense benefits from being hand ground in a mortar and pestle. Grind the ingredients one at a time, awakening them as you go:

> Trees of this place, I call you to attention. DESCRIBE SITUATION. Entangle the land in your roots. DESCRIBE DESIRED OUTCOME. Artemisia, beloved defender of the wild places, DESCRIBE SITUATION. Awaken the land to fight. DESCRIBE DESIRED OUTCOME. Cloves, little nails, little warriors, DESCRIBE SITUATION, lend me your strength. Landcestors, martyrs, may your bravery awaken once more. DESCRIBE SITUATION. Help me! DESCRIBE DESIRED OUTCOME. Despoiler, you have seen the wages of your sin. The

time has come to make reparations! DESCRIBE SITUATION. Earn your redemption now! DESCRIBE DESIRED OUTCOME.

Phase Two: Enchant the Nails

Once the incense is compounded, gather your nails. For a temporary hold—which is what I recommend in most cases—use wood spikes made from fallen wood gathered as close as possible to the land in question. Eventually, as the spikes decay back into the land, the spell will be released. This is the best option. You can always respike it every few years if you want to keep it going. On the other hand, for a permanent effect, you can also use metal nails or, ideally, railroad spikes. In order to unweave this spell, you will have to remove the spikes. I recommend this only in cases of natural land preservation and conservation in places like parks and wildlife reserves.

Why do I recommend against it in other cases? A story: When we were about fifteen, my best friend's grandmother was about to lose her cottage. My friend and I, who were just starting to learn witchcraft together, spiked the property, and she managed to keep it. Almost twenty years later, that same friend and I were trying to buy it from her grandmother, to keep it in the family. Despite her grandmother being entirely on board, we hit one logistical nightmare after another before we remembered the spikes. We spent a very cold, wet night hunting twenty-year-old spikes in the rain. We only found three, and even for us, both of whom had been seriously studying and practicing witchcraft for decades, it took some doing to unweave the spell enough to sell it "in family" with that one spike still in. Lesson learned: "until iron decays" is too long for most spells. Use wooden spikes, and keep track of where you put them.

Before you begin, write a very clear and specific petition, outlining the particulars of what you want. Prepare a working space where you can howl out loud without being interrupted. Enter into magical space, time, and consciousness. Pick up the spikes. Stoke a red-hot fury inside yourself. Get *mad* that people are attempting to drive you off your home—or despoil the land, or whatever it is you're mad about. Feel the red-hot fire tighten in your chest, but sit very quietly and still. Do not allow it to escape. When you cannot bear it any longer, force the feeling down your arms and howl as loudly as you can, feeling the fire fill the spikes. If using metal spikes, put a lit charcoal directly on top of them, and burn the incense while you read aloud your petition. If using wooden spikes, pass them through the incense smoke while you read. Exit magical space, time, and consciousness and immediately go wash your hands and drink some water. If you are having trouble shaking the rage, hit a boxing bag or take a run, etc., until you have exhausted it. If you routinely have trouble shaking off the magical vibes after spellwork, that is a sign that you would benefit from a stronger meditation practice.

Phase Three: Plant the Spikes

Investigate the location you'd like to spike. Ideally, you'll be able to plant a spike at every corner of the property. However, in some cases that is not possible. If you do not have access to the corners, find a suitable location you can spike. I do not recommend spiking trees, even to prevent logging. It can maim or kill the worker doing the logging, who is not the enemy. Their masters are the enemy, and that worker is just cannon fodder to them. Some options are spiking on either side of the main gate, spiking the road leading up to the site, spiking around a prominent sign or statue, or spiking at the exact center of the site. In extremity, you can even make a sort of location poppet out of a map and spike that, but it's much less effective. If possible, pass the spikes off to someone who has better access to the site. I would certainly never recommend you trespass, but if you're sneaking around at night, remember to stay safe. The actual spiking is short and sweet. Just pound the spikes into the ground, and say something like: "May the land and trees bear witness! No development here!!" I like to go clockwise around the boundary of the property, starting and ending by the main entrance, but it doesn't really matter.

FETCHING CHARM

This spell is designed to force someone to contact you. Like all nonconsensual magic, it should be deployed carefully and only in appropriate situations. This spell will cause a person to contact you, but does not guarantee the results of that contact. For most purposes, it should be combined with other spellwork. This spell is strongly informed by PGM VII 593-619 and uses a very classic technique in malefica: slandering the gods in your adversary's name. The original spell calls for a lamp, not painted red, with seven wicks made from rope from a sunken ship, which are written on with myrrh ink and fed wormwood seeds. This version, which uses incense instead of an oil lamp, simplifies the procedure, but expands it slightly by repeating it over several nights. I have also updated the specifics of the slander to modern sensibility.

2 parts wormwood

1 part myrrh

Print a picture of the target, and attach any personal concerns. Put your incense holder or bowl on top of the picture, light the incense, and speak the following formula. As you say each blasphemy, drop a single whole clove onto the incense. Take note of which ones pop.

> *I call upon you, lords, great gods, who shine in this present hour, on this day, for the sake of NAME, the ungodly.*
>
> *They, NAME, have said IAO is a spineless coward.*
>
> *They, NAME, have said Adonai was cast out of heaven because of his violent rage.*
>
> *They, NAME, have said Sabaoth cries like a little baby: wah, wah, wah.*
>
> *They, NAME, not I, have said that Pagoure is an unnatural monster.*
>
> *They, NAME, have said that Marmorouth has been shamefully defeated.*
>
> *They, NAME, have said IAEO could not be trusted with the holy ark.*
>
> *They, NAME, have said that Michael is a sellout bootlicker.*
>
> *It is not I, NAME, but they, NAME, who say such impious things. Cause them to be distressed, enflamed, unable to sleep until they contact me, for I am your loyal servant.*

The more cloves pop, the closer they are to contacting you. Repeat the spell nightly until you get seven cloves to pop.

CHILL OUT!

This incense and the spell that follows it are designed to defuse anger and encourage negotiation, compromise, and forgiveness from all who interact with you. They are especially effective against employers, cops, teachers, or others in a position of power over the caster. They are much more effective when cast on a specific person, whose name you know, but the spell can also be cast on more abstract targets like "the justice system." Expect this kind of largely metaphorical magic to get largely metaphorical results.

> 2 parts pine or another resin
>
> 3 parts mugwort
>
> 1 part vervain
>
> 1 part clover flower or lavender

A Freezer Spell to Restrain Anger

This spell, which is very vaguely based on PGM X 24-35, is best performed on a Saturday night, ideally in the hour of the moon while the moon wanes, but any other time works too.

YOU WILL NEED

> Incense for burning—and extra for packing the box
>
> A poppet of the target
>
> A small box the poppet fits inside
>
> Aluminum foil
>
> Glue
>
> A kitchen towel or other fluffy piece of fabric
>
> A ballpoint pen
>
> Lead fishing weights (You can get these at any outdoor store. I like the
>   kind shaped like teardrops for this, but it doesn't really matter.)
>
> Black ribbon
>
> A freezer or snowbank
>
> A glass of lemonade
>
> Some salt

Before entering magical space, time, and consciousness, prepare the poppet. Set the poppet aside, and carefully line the inside of the box in foil. Cut a piece of foil just big enough to put inside the lid. Fold the kitchen towel to make a padded surface, put the foil on it, and use a ballpoint pen to carefully emboss the following design into the foil. If you pierce the foil, or mess it up in some other way, throw it out and start again.

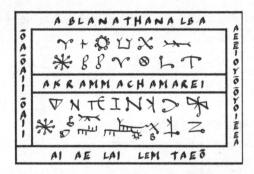

Now that everything is ready, light the incense and enter magical space, time, and consciousness. Baptize the poppet, and place it in the box. Cover it with the foil talisman, with the impressions you made facedown. Conjure within yourself a feeling of heavy, cold, and drowsiness, mixed with a vaguely depressed ennui. Even if you wanted to hurt someone, it just feels so hard and pointless. Really, doing almost anything just seems very hard. You're so tired. Once you have that feeling, push it out of your hands and into the lead weights, and then place them on top of the foil. Fill the box with loose incense, put the lid on, and use the black ribbon to tie it closed. Label the bottom of the box, so that when you find the box years from now, you don't have to open it to remember what it is. Put the whole box, tied shut, into the freezer, or push it deep within a snowbank. Exit magical space, time, and consciousness. Go wash your hands, then drink the lemonade and sprinkle a little salt on top of your head. If you are still having trouble shaking the heaviness, take a bath in hot salt water.

SHUT THE F*CK UP!

This incense is designed to stop people from slandering you, although it can also be deployed in other circumstances, such as to prevent a coconspirator from confessing. It can also be used to good effect in local political magic to disrupt an opponent's propaganda. While the spell is designed to be applied to a single human target, with some creative sorcery poppets can also be made for more abstract "people" like corporations.

3 parts artemisia (Wormwood is preferable.)

2 parts myrrh

1 part cloves

Just a pinch of Virginia creeper, ivy, morning glory, bindweed, or any other aggressive vine

YOU WILL NEED

Incense

A photo of your target's face, blown up large

Personal concerns, attached to the photo

Needle with red thread

About an hour, ideally on a Saturday when the moon is dark

WHAT TO DO

As with all malefica, it's best to write yourself a script, so you don't let your emotions carry you away. Below is a sample. You should write your own based on your specific situation. Once you are happy with your script, light the incense and enter into magical space, time, and consciousness. Call to mind everything you know about the target, and overlap that mental image over the photo. Wave the photo over the incense, and speak to it, saying something like:

Creature of paper, I, NAME, breathe life into you. You are now NAME, the child of NAME and NAME, who lives at ADDRESS, and DESCRIPTION. What happens to you happens to them.

Put the photo down, and put your dominant hand, in a fist, on your breast-bone. Push on it with your other hand. Stoke a red heart flame of rage in your chest, and push it into your dominant hand, both through your chest and by running it down both arms. When your hand is hot with power, pick up the needle, and slowly sew the lips of the poppet shut, reading your script, which might go something like:

NAME, I sew you shut. No longer will you be able to talk trash about me. If you speak against me, you will choke, your lungs filling with smoke, your throat on fire with pain. Etc., etc. . . .

When you've poured out all the energy, wave the poppet through the incense smoke a final time, and then pour water over the incense charcoal until it is completely cold. Use your dominant-hand index finger to paint a large *X* over the poppet's face with the wet incense ash. When you are done, carefully wash your hands. Take a shower or bath before you go to sleep. Repeat the spell for at least three, but no more than seven, nights.

DO WHAT I SAY!

This incense is of a category usually called dominating, compelling, or commanding work. It's designed to force someone to do something they don't want to do. Generally, I recommend against this kind of work, but it can be necessary in some circumstances. This is gentler than many formulas, rarely causing harm. One traditional use is for debt collection, as in the spell provided below.

  1 part dragon's blood

  2 parts cedar

  1 part spicebush or allspice

  1 part licorice root

  1 part calamus (sweet flag) root

A Spell to Collect a Debt

This spell will compel a person to pay a debt they owe you, if they are able to do so. If they genuinely cannot afford to pay, this spell will likely fail. You can't get blood from a turnip.

YOU WILL NEED

  Incense—a lot of it

  A contract or other document acknowledging the debt (It is *much* better if
    the document contains their signature.)

  A photo of the debtor, sized to fit the candle

Scissors

A black taper candle

14 extra-long straight pins

WHAT TO DO

◆ Cut the head off the photo to make a sort of mask for the candle.

◆ Carve the debtor's name into the candle with a pin.

◆ Use a pin to attach the face to the candle to make a sort of doll.

◆ Light the incense.

◆ Baptize the candle as your debtor, and fumigate it in the incense.

◆ Roll the contract around the candle, attaching it with pins, while . . .

◆ Speaking from your heart, from a place of cold anger, say
   something like:

◆ Creature of wax, who are NAME, I constrain you, I compel you,
   I command you to pay what is owed to me now. As these pins
   pierce you, so too are you pierced by guilt. Until you pay me, you
   will have no rest. I pierce you with this pin; it will sting you until
   you pay.

GO AWAY!

Since time out of mind, getting rid of bad neighbors has been a classic form
of magic. I suspect spells to drive away "those people" were common trade
for witches in every culture that has ever been. Certainly, such spells are
common in most ancient compendiums of folk magic. In modern American
folk magic, such work is often called hot foot work, a term which origi-
nates in Hoodoo.

   This type of magic tends to take three tactics: (1) appealing directly to
the spirits of the house or land to evict them, (2) intimidating and scaring
them into leaving, and (3) making elsewhere more attractive to them. For
the most part, I advocate doing all three, which is what we'll be under-
taking in the following, used in conjunction with the incense below. In

addition to this spell, the incense can be used in any type of "Go Away!" or hot foot–style workings.

GO AWAY INCENSE

2 parts resin of any type but hyper-local is best

1 part rosemary, keeping the needles whole to better rankle them

1 part whole black peppercorns

1 part crushed dried wasps (optional)

1 part coarse rock salt

1 part dirt from their threshold

BEFORE BEGINNING

♦ Discover their names.

♦ Write a sort of "list of charges" explaining everything that is wrong with your neighbors. These should be things that are objectively wrong, like littering or being cruel. Ideally, cite specific crimes: "On the 3rd of April, they ran over my dog." "They always park in my handicapped space." Or "They shoveled their walk onto mine last week."

♦ Write another list, as a sort of character reference. Why should the Land like you better? As before, try to cite specific incidents. "Do I not always shovel not just my walk, but also my elderly neighbors?" "I give you milk and cake whenever the moon is full." "I cleared out those invasive weeds, and have planted seven trees." Or "I do not eat meat, and I recycle all my cans." Etc.

♦ Prepare an especially elaborate offering. If possible, plant a tree. Evergreens with sharp needles are especially good for this work.

♦ Prepare or acquire a hot foot–style incense, charcoal, and a censer. Minimally, you can use whole black peppercorns. *Do not* use ground pepper. If you need to be stealthy, carefully empty a filtered cigarette, grind the incense very fine, mix a tiny bit into the tobacco, and carefully restuff the cigarette. This trick should only be done with martial incenses, and others where tobacco is "on topic." *Do not* smoke the cigarette, but light it and then wave it around like you're frustrated. In dire straits, cigarettes are perfectly acceptable incense for most combative magic—and also necromancy, and lots of other things.

THE RITUAL

♦ Astrological timing isn't important, but the wind, if it blows, should be blowing from you to them. It's best to do this work outside, but it can be done indoors. Open a window.

♦ Enter into magical space, time, and consciousness by any method.

♦ Ground out through your navel and into the center of the Earth. Ideally, travel by way of a local tree's roots, but any path is fine.

♦ Greet the Land in your usual fashion, and make the offering. Imagine it multiplying out to infinity as you do so. Save a final dessert for the end; sugar cookies are especially good for this.

♦ Remind it what a good tenant you have been. Use the letter of reference you wrote.

♦ Ask if there is anything you can do for it. If it's simple, do it, but you don't have to agree to whatever is asked. Do not continue until something you can do for the Land comes to mind. When in doubt, plant a native tree.

♦ Having done a favor for them, ask them for a favor in return. You would like the spirits of the Land to reach out and find the place in the world that is best for the neighbors and to send them on their way to that place. Call them out by name. Remind the Land what is wrong with them. Read the list of charges, and ask the Land to pass sentence and exile them.

♦ Ensure that the wind, if it blows, blows from where you are toward the offending neighbor.

- Stand downwind of the incense, and light it and the charges. If the wind is not blowing, blow the smoke toward the neighbors.

- Say something that sounds appropriately fairy-tale-ish telling them to go away in the name of the Land. In English, we might say: "Hie thee hence! Hie thee hence! The Gentry say Get Thee Thither!"

- Rejoice in your friendship with the Land. Dance and play with it. That last dessert I had you save from the offering? Split it with the Land now, being sure to also offer your uniquely human experience of it; let them share in your tasting of it. This is a thing they crave, but you have to save it for a special treat; it's not really very good for you. (This is what people are talking about when they say things like "eating fairy food" or "eating goblin fruit.") Abide in the communion for a little while, and then politely say goodbye. *Do not* fall asleep in fairyland. It's best to just stay on your feet.

- Put out the incense, if it is still burning, by pouring clean water over it.

- Make a paste or potion of the ashes and some water, and contrive to touch the neighbor's doorknob with it, if possible. If not, pour it out onto the Land, and instruct it to travel below the Earth to them.

- Repeat every night for seven nights. If the wind is wrong, perform the spell, but do not light the incense.

- Ideally, the wind should blow strongly toward them on the last night. If you get a night with very strong favorable winds, you might choose to end there, even if you're not yet to seven.

BREAK UP

This spell, modeled on one from the Greek Magical Papyri, is designed to break a couple up. With minor adaptations it can also be used to get someone fired or to separate them from another type of organization. The original spell relies on leaving a pot of stinky fermented fish on the couple's doorstep for its noxious power; we'll use this incense instead. This incense doesn't store well; make a small batch for onetime use. Alternatively, you can make a bigger batch without the anchovy paste, and mix that in just before use.

    1 part myrrh, powdered, for the depths of the underworld

    1 part cedarwood, mostly just to add body and extend the burn time

    2 parts wormwood for pungency and its malefic attributes

    3 parts onion and garlic peels to bring tears to the eyes

    Anchovy paste to bind and make it stink

TO PERFORM THE SPELL, YOU WILL NEED

    A large bowl, half full of dirt

    Incense charcoal (Do not use an electric burner for this spell.)

    A small candle

    A lighter

    A glass of muddy water

    A photo of the couple together (A printout is good.)

    A black marker

    Hatred and fury

    About an hour

WHAT TO DO

◆ Begin by setting up the charcoal in the bowl. Do not light it yet.

◆ Turn the photo over and write the following magic words on the back, exactly as they appear below:

ʻΙΑΙΑ ʻΙΑΚΟΥΒ ΙΑΙ ʻΙΩ ʻΕΡΒΗΘ ʻΙΩ ΠΑΚΕΡΒΗΘ

ʻΙΩ ΒΟΛΧΟΣΗΘ, ΒΑΣΔΟΥΜΑ ΠΑΤΑΥΝΑΞ,

ΑΠΟΨΟΣΕΣΡΩ ΑΤΑΦ ΘΑΒΡΑΟΥ ΗΩ ΥΑΥΥΑΒΡΑ ΒΩΡΑΡΑ

ΑΡΟΒΡΕΙΥΑ ΒΟΛΧΟΣΗΘ, ΚΟΚΚΟΛΟΙΠΤΟΛΗ ΡΑΜΒΙΘΝΙΨ

◆ Turn the photo over, and light the incense and candle.

- Recall to mind your hate and fury for the couple. Feel the desire to hurt them well up in you.

- Focus your feeling into the photo, while waving it over the incense.

- Speak from your heart, saying something like:

  I call upon you, god of the empty air, of the wild places. You are terrible, invisible, and mighty. You afflict the earth with pestilence and shake the universe to its foundations. You love disturbances and hate stability. You scatter the clouds from one another, so there is only baking sun. So too, bring strife and war to NAME, child of NAMES, and NAME, child of NAMES. Make between them odious enmity, just like Typhon and Isis had. Strong spirit, very powerful one, perform your mighty acts!

- You may wish to repeat it several times, building up fury. When you reach a crescendo . . .

- Tear the photo in half, separating the couple, and carefully burn both halves over the incense.

- When the photo is completely reduced to ash . . .

- Pour the muddy water over it, putting out the fire and producing a mud paste.

- Ideally, smear the paste across the couple's threshold if they live together. Dispose of the rest of it far from your house, ideally in a metal dumpster.

- Take a shower, washing very carefully, and end with pouring a large pitcher of salt water over your head.

Interpreting Ancient Recipes

MANY ANCIENT INCENSE recipes survive into our day. However, even with the full text of the recipe on hand, it can be difficult to get from that to a modern recipe. Often ancient languages use the same word for broad categories of plants; this is particularly true for texts not written in the indigenous language of their region, such as the PGM's somewhat slapdash use of Greek names for Egyptian and Levantine plants.

Moreover, even when we think we can determine what is being referenced, most plants used in incense were—and still are—luxury trade goods. Where there's a profit to be made, we humans domesticate plants aggressively. We discussed this in the marijuana section, but that is just one extreme example. Our herbs, generally, are not the same as those of our ancestors. Although our ancestors did not have quite our modern knowledge of domestication, they were still highly skilled for their time and had thousands of years over which to ply that craft.

Then once we think we've narrowed down the ingredients, there can still be confusing translation issues. Ancient measuring systems are not always easy to interpret. This is particularly true in texts like the PGM, which were not intended for publication. Just like grandma, those magicians generally measured their recipes in pinches, bits, and "good portions." There are also subtler problems; bulleted lists are a very new invention. The lack of punctuation in many ancient written languages sometimes makes it hard to determine which measurements apply to which ingredient. As you will see in this chapter, this is especially pronounced in very ancient texts such as the Torah.

Finally, almost all ancient recipes were intended to be crafted in a very small geographic region with fresh, local ingredients. The same incense would have been prepared differently in every region, and by every temple, and those personal recipes were closely guarded secrets. For all these reasons and more, I would never claim to provide authentic recipes for ancient incense, any more than I would claim my spanakopita recipe is the only authentic one. In this chapter, I'll interpret several ancient recipes for modern use. As always, you should consider these as examples for your own experimentation. We'll work our way backward in time, gaining interpretive skill as we go.

The Sacred Magic of Abramelin the Mage

15TH CENTURY CE, GERMANY

The Sacred Book of Abramelin is a German grimoire, which claims to have been written by Abraham of Worms in 1458. Although that cannot be confirmed, most experts agree that it most likely did originate in a German Jewish community in the 15th century. The book chronicles the travels of Abraham from Germany to Egypt, where he meets a magician named Abramelin, who teaches him the magic contained within the book. The book is distinguished from other similar grimoires primarily because it provides an elaborate initiatory ritual that promised "knowledge and conversation" with the "Holy Guardian Angel." In book two, toward the end of chapter eleven, there appears the following incense recipe, which has become very popular for all types of angel work, largely owing to Aleister Crowley's fondness for it.

Until recently, the most popular formulation was based on S. L. MacGregor Mathers's 1898 translation of a late French manuscript. A more recent translation by George Dehn and Steven Guth presents another version from older German manuscripts. Both versions appear to be simplified variants of ketoret, which I prefer to either of these. We'll discuss ketoret at the end of this chapter.

MATHERS'S VERSION

The perfume shall be made thus: Take of incense in tears one part; of stacte half a part; of lign aloes a quarter of a part and not being able to get this wood you shall take that of cedar, or of rose, or of citron, or any other odoriferous wood. You shall reduce all these ingredients into a very fine powder, mix them well together; and keep the same in a box or other convenient vessel.

Keeping the ratios the same, we can scale up as we interpret the ingredients with modern equivalents. *Stacte* (στακτή) means "ooze" in Greek and indicates resin, usually myrrh. We'll discuss it further in the section about ketoret.

- 4 parts frankincense
- 2 parts myrrh
- 1 part aloeswood or any other aromatic wood (Personally, I like cedar.)

DEHN AND GUTH VERSION

Take equal amounts of balm, gummy galbanum, and pure storax. If you cannot get balm, use cedar or aloe or other pleasantly-smelling woods. Mix the ingredients together as a powder. Keep it in a clean container.

- 1 part balsam or an aromatic wood
- 1 part galbanum
- 1 part storax

Sefer Raziel, Book Three

13TH CENTURY CE, ASHKENAZ

Sefer Raziel h'Malakh (ראלמה לאיזר רפס), or The Book of the Angel of the Secrets of El, is a medieval Jewish Solomonic-style grimoire most likely compiled in the 13th century, but drawn from older sources. Book three of the text discusses incense, providing recommendations for each day of the week. A loose translation follows.

> The Angel taught Adam how to make incenses: Incenses are a confection of good scent with which you shall fumigate and thus please Creation, and therefore will you attain whatever you will. They should be made of precious things, which you will learn, pleasing of scent and altogether clean. When you do this, you too must be clean and without any pollution. . . . The Creator spoke to Moses, saying, "Make incense and fumigate the hill (Mt. Sinai) when you wish to speak with me. So Solomon said that suffumigations and sacrifice and balm make open the gates of the ether and of the fire, and of all the other heavens. By such suffumigation a man may see heavenly things . . . There are seven heavens and seven stars and seven days in the week . . .
>
> The first incense of Saturday must be of all good things, and good-smelling roots, such as costus and storax.
>
> Incense of Sunday is frankincense, mastic, musk, and such. All other good resins of pleasing scent are good.
>
> Incense of Monday is myrtle leaves and bay laurel and (other) good-smelling leaves.
>
> Incense of Tuesday is sandalwoods, red, black, and white and all such trees, and aloeswood and cypress.
>
> Incense of Wednesday is made of all barks, such as cinnamon, cassia, laurel bark, and mace.
>
> Incense of Thursday is nutmeg, clove, citron peel, and the dried pulverized rind of oranges, and all other fruits of good odors.
>
> Incense of Friday is rose, violets, crocus (saffron), and all other sweet-smelling flowers.
>
> . . . And Hermes said the supreme incense is cinnamon, aloeswood, mastic, crocus (saffron), costus, mace, and myrtle. . . . Each of the planets has a part in it.

As a modern version of this supreme incense, I recommend:

- 1 part cinnamon or cassia
- 2 parts sandalwood or cedar
- 1 part mastic
- 2 parts orris root (*Saussurea costus* is a type of thistle whose roots were used in ancient perfumery. Today, the species is severely threatened. Orris root has a similar floral smell and fixative action, so I've chosen to use it instead.)
- 1 part mace or nutmeg
- 1 part myrtle
- 1 string saffron per burn

Codex Sangallensis 761

EARLY 9TH CENTURY CE, SWITZERLAND

The Abbey Library of St. Gall in Switzerland houses a large library of medieval texts. Among these is #761, a medical text that contains a collection of nearly fifty medicinal remedies. The final entry is simply titled "Thimiama" (Incense). No instructions are given for preparation or use. The text reads: *Thimiama : cozumber – 3, aloeswood, ambergris – 3 denarii, confita, camphor – 1 denarius, musk – 1 denarius.*

Most of these ingredients are clear, but *cozumber* and *confita* are a mystery. Some scholars suggest that cozumber was a precious aromatic gum used in the church. In my interpretation below, I use amber, based on the slight similarity in sound. Aloeswood is another name for agarwood. As we discussed in the chapter on aromatic woods, it is difficult to source ethically. I have substituted sandalwood. Ambergris is a waxy substance produced in the digestive systems of sperm whales. For pretty obvious reasons, it has been largely replaced by synthetic substitutes. To provide a similarly rich and decadent woodsy scent, I've chosen cypress and clary sage.

The word *confita* is possibly derived from the Latin roots *con* and *facio* which mean "mixed together." Given the context, I would expect this recipe to include either frankincense or myrrh, but it calls for neither.

For this reason, I've guessed that confita might mean "mixed resins" or "standard church incense mix." Camphor is clear and requires no substitution. Musk here indicates a glandular secretion of the musk deer, which was a common element in perfumery from antiquity until the 19th century, when it was largely replaced with synthetic scents. I have substituted the seeds of *Abelmoschus moschatus*, sometimes called musk seed, rose mallow, or musk ambrette. They can be found online or in some Indian grocers and health stores. I do not especially care for this scent, so I have cut the amount called for.

The amounts in the original recipe are measured in denarii; one denarius is about 4.5 grams. It is not entirely clear what amounts are being called for. I interpret it as calling for three parts cozumber, three parts of mixed aloeswood and ambergris, one part mixed confita and camphor, and one part musk. Based largely on experimentation, I've developed the following modern interpretation:

6 parts amber

4 parts sandalwood

3 parts cypress wood

1 part clary sage

6 parts mixed resins (I like 2 parts each of frankincense, myrrh, and mastic.)

2 parts camphor

1 part musk seed

Eighth Book of Moses

4TH CENTURY CE, GRECO-ROMAN EGYPT

The Eighth Book of Moses, which is also called PGM XIII, provides several incense recipes. In the beginning, it offers the following suggestions for planetary incenses:

Kronos (Saturn) styrax "for it is heavy and fragrant"

Zeus (Jupiter) malabathron

Ares (Mars) kostos

Helios (Sun) frankincense

Aphrodite (Venus) spikenard

Hermes (Mercury) cassia

Selene (Moon) myrrh

Next, it describes an incense of the seven flowers of the seven stars: marjoram, lily, lotus, erephyllinon, narcissus (aka daffodil), gillyflower (aka wallflower), and rose. All are easily identified except erephyllinon (ἐρεφύλλινον), which has stumped scholars. Its place in the list indicates it is a solar flower. The related word ἑρπύλλινον indicates a type of thyme, so thyme flower is what I would use.

Kyphi

2ND CENTURY BCE, PTOLEMAIC EGYPT

Kyphi (κῦφι) is the Greek name for traditional Egyptian incense. The word does not describe a particular recipe, but rather a broad class of similar mixtures. Many ancient recipes survive, both Egyptian and Greek. Most of them are built around mixed resins, galangal, juniper berries, and cinnamon. Most versions are bound with a syrup made by soaking raisins in wine until fully rehydrated—this takes several days—and then blending to a thick paste. Often, honey is added. You can also experiment with using date honey, which is available in any Middle Eastern grocer.

My version, below, is most closely modeled on one inscribed into the walls of the great temple of Horus at Edfu, but is a mixture of several ancient recipes.

8 parts cypress wood

8 parts juniper berries

6 parts frankincense

6 parts myrrh

4 parts mastic

4 parts pine resin

4 parts cinnamon

2 parts cardamom

2 parts galangal

2 parts sweet flag

2 parts rooibos tea

1 part lemongrass

1 part mint

Grind all the ingredients to a very fine powder, and set aside about a quarter of it. Slowly add date honey to the larger portion until a sticky dough is formed. Roll it into balls. I like to make balls of mixed sizes, so I can choose how much to burn at a time. Roll each ball in the reserved powder until it's not sticky. Allow the incense balls to sit out overnight so they dry out a little, and then give them another coat of powdered resin on the outside if they're still sticky. Although this incense can be stored at cool room temperature, I prefer to refrigerate it to preserve freshness.

Ketoret

HEBREW, SECOND MILLENNIUM BCE

The Hebrew word *ketoret* (קְטֹרֶת) simply means "incense," rather than indicating any specific recipe. However, in the context of modern Anglophone magic, ketoret usually refers to incenses intended to replicate the offering incense of Solomon's Temple. The thirtieth chapter of שמות (Shemot) describes the construction of an altar for incense offerings. This chapter includes a recipe for holy anointing oil and warnings against its use for profane purposes. At the end of the chapter, the recipe for holy incense is given, and again the reader is warned not to make it for selfish reasons, but only to use it for holy purposes:

וַיֹּאמֶר יְהוָה אֶל־מֹשֶׁה קַח־לְךָ סַמִּים נָטָף וּ שְׁחֵלֶת וְחֶלְבְּנָה סַמִּים וּלְבֹנָה זַכָּה בַּד בְּבַד יִהְיֶה׃

And HaShem said to Moses: Take sweet spices—נטף and שחלת, and galbanum—these sweet spices with pure frankincense: of each there should be a like weight.

Even more so than the other recipes we've discussed, this one is difficult to interpret. It is almost one thousand years older than any of the recipes we've discussed. In addition to both translation and evolution issues, there are also millennia of complex religious exegesis surrounding the recipe.

Opinions differ on how many ingredients are listed. As you can see from my translation above, I believe that the sweet spices in question are the three ingredients listed next. Others disagree, and add cinnamon, cassia, and other sweet spices in addition to those explicitly listed. That is a reasonable concern; my recipe is all resins, and contains no actual spices. For a variety of numerological reasons, some commentators favor recipes with eleven ingredients, and several such recipes are known. Of the four ingredients explicitly listed, only two, frankincense and galbanum, are easy to translate.

The other two are less clear. In this verse, נָטָף (*nataf*) is usually translated with the Greek word στακτή (*stacte*). נָטָף means "droplet" and στακτή means "goo," and both clearly refer to some kind of sap or resin in this context. However, it is unclear what type of resin is being called for—or, perhaps, different resins were used at different times. Most ancient commentators believed נָטָף to be a special type of myrrh, although there are other opinions. When I formulate this incense, I use myrrh or occasionally myrrh and storax.

The other, תלחש (*shecheleth*), normally means "roar" or "lion-like" or "peel away." However, it is related to a family of Hebrew words that cluster around meaning "black" and also some Syrian words that mean "tear" or "distillate," which could perhaps imply a resin from Syria, possibly benzoin or storax. In Greek, תלחש was most often translated as ονυξ (*onycha*), which usually means "onyx-like" or "black," but can also mean "similar to veins in stone," as well as "fingernail" or "claw." Based on this reading, another possible option is a type of sea snail called a "devil's fingernail." The whelks have a sort of hard lid, like a fingernail. When properly processed before being burned, these produce a very pleasant smell and were used in incense in antiquity. I (and many others) are skeptical of this interpretation, as (1) sea snails are not kosher, and (2) they are definitely not a "spice." The Talmud, on the other hand, suggests that onycha comes from a bush. Is there perhaps a black resin that comes from a bush that grows in Syria? There is! It's called labdanum, and it's produced by several species of rockrose. This is what I use when I make ketoret.

With those interpretations, the recipe is:

1 part galbanum

1 part myrrh

1 part labdanum

3 parts frankincense

Notes

1. Yoshinori Shichida, Takahiro Yamashita, Hiroo Imai, and Takushi Kishida, *Evolution and Senses: Opsins, Bitter Taste, and Olfaction* (New York: Springer, 2013).
2. Jamie Morgan, "Womb with a View: Sensory Development in Utero," *UT Southwestern Medical Center*, August 1, 2017. *utswmed.org*.
3. Ibid.
4. Ibid.
5. Ibid.
6. Luca Turin, *The Secret of Scent: Adventures in Perfume and the Science of Smell* (New York: Harper Perennial, 2007).
7. Ibid.
8. Ibid.
9. Ibid.
10. Ibid.
11. Diane Ackerman, *A Natural History of the Senses* (New York: Knopf Doubleday Publishing Group, 2011).
12. C. S. Sell, *Chemistry and the Sense of Smell* (Hoboken, NJ: Wiley, 2014).
13. Emma Flatt, "Spices, Smells and Spells: The Use of Olfactory Substances in the Conjuring of Spirits," *South Asian Studies* 32, no. 1 (April 2016): 3–21.
14. Winai Sayorwan, Nijsiri Ruangrungsi, Teerut Piriyapunyporn, Tapnee Hongratanaworakit, Naiphinich Kotchabhakdi, and Vorasith Siripornpanich, "Effects of Inhaled Rosemary Oil on Subjective Feelings and Activities of the Nervous System," *Scientia Pharmaceutica* 81, no. 2 (April-June 2013): 531–42.
15. Kevin Bradford, "The Use of Scents to Influence Consumers: The Sense of Using Scents to Make Cents," *Journal of Business Ethics* 90 (November 2009): 141–53.
16. Brian Handwerk, "In Some Ways, Your Sense of Smell Is Actually Better Than a Dog's," *Smithsonian Magazine*, May 2017. *www.smithsonianmag.com*.
17. Ibid.
18. Sell, *Chemistry and the Sense of Smell*.
19. Kjeld Nielsen, *Incense in Ancient Israel* (Leiden, The Netherlands: Brill Academic Publishing, 2014), 3.
20. David Michael Stoddart, *The Scented Ape: The Biology and Culture of Human Odour* (Cambridge, UK: Cambridge University Press, 1990), 169.
21. Henry Smith Williams, *The Historians' History of the World: A Comprehensive Narrative of the Rise and Development of Nations from the Earliest Times, Volumes 1–2* (Encyclopaedia Britannica, 1907), 226.
22. I. E. S. Edwards, C. J. Gadd, and N. G. L. Hammond, eds., *The Cambridge Ancient History* (Cambridge, UK: Cambridge University Press, 1969), 330.
23. Edward Godfrey Cuthbert Frederic Atchley, *A History of the Use of Incense in Divine Worship* (London and New York: Longmans, Green and Co., 1909).
24. David Rollason, *Early Medieval Europe 300–1050: A Guide for Studying and Teaching*, second edition (London: Routledge, 2018). This book has no page numbers, but the relevant discussion is in part IV, chapter 9, in the section labeled "Trade with the Arabic Caliphate" under the topic heading "Spices."

25. Gus W. Van Beek, "Frankincense and Myrrh in Ancient South Arabia," *Journal of the American Oriental Society* 78, no. 3 (July-September 1958): 141–52. *www.jstor.org*.

26. Herodotus, *The History of Herodotus*, translated by George Rawlinson (London: John Murray, 1858*)*, *mit.edu*. 2:75, 1–4.

27. Mulugeta Lemenih and Demel Teketay, "Frankincense and Myrrh Resources of Ethiopia: II. Medicinal and Industrial Uses," *SINET: Ethiopian Journal of Science* 26, no. 2 (2003): 161–72. *semanticscholar.org*.

28. Danielle M. Strebel, Andrew J. Fangel, Tony M. Wolfe, and Emily J. Mason, "Anxiolytic and Anti-Depressant Effects of *Boswellia* Extract on CD1 *Mus musculus*," *BIOS* 85, no. 2 (May 2014): 79–85. *doi.org*.

29. I. Epstein, ed., *Tractate Sanhedrin*, translated by Jacob Shachter and H. Freedman (London: Soncino Press, 1987), Sanhedrin 43a.

30. Pearce Paul Creasman and Kei Yamamoto, "The African Incense Trade and Its Impacts in Pharaonic Egypt," *African Archeological Review* 36 (August 2019): 347–65. *doi.org*.

31. Colin Schultz, "There's More to Frankincense and Myrrh Than Meets the Eye," *Smithsonian Magazine*, December 24, 2014. *www.smithsonianmag.com*.

32. Karl Preisendanz, *Papyri Graecae Magicae, Volume 1* (Leipzig, Germany: Teubner, 1928). *doi.org*. From this point on, Greek Magical Papyri will be abbreviated, as is customary, as PGM.

33. Wendy Makoons Geniusz, *Our Knowledge Is Not Primitive: Decolonizing Botanical Anishinaabe Teachings (The Iroquois and Their Neighbors)* (Syracuse, NY: Syracuse University Press, 2009), 73.

34. Jacques Rousseau, "Le Folklore Botanique De Caughnawaga," *Contributions de l'Institut botanique l'Universite de Montreal* 55 (1945): 7–72. Here p. 35.

35. Melvin Randolph Gilmore, *Some Chippewa Uses of Plants* (Ann Arbor, MI: University of Michigan Press, 1933), 34.

36. Huron H. Smith, "Ethnobotany of the Forest Potawatomi Indians," *Bulletin of the Public Museum of the City of Milwaukee* 7 (1933): 1–230. Here p. 70–71.

37. Paul Hamel and Mary Ulmer Chiltoskey, *Cherokee Plants and Their Uses: A 400 Year History* (Sylva, NC: Herald Publishing Company, 1975), 28.

38. Shelly Katheren Kraft, "Recent Changes in the Ethnobotany of Standing Rock Indian Reservation." (M.A. thesis, University of North Dakota, Grand Forks, 1990), 30.

39. Francis Hapgood Elmore, *Ethnobotany of the Navajo* (Santa Fe, NM: School of American Research, 1944), 20. *babel.hathitrust.org*.

40. Gilmore, *Some Chippewa Uses of Plants*, 73.

41. D. C. Watts, *Dictionary of Plant Lore* (Cambridge, MA: Academic Press, 2007), 309.

42. Odin (human author unknown), Nine Herbs Charm, mid-10th century, translated by Wikisource, lines 1–6. *en.wikisource.org*.

43. Halina Ekiert, Joanna Pajor, Paweł Klin, Agnieszka Rzepiela, Halina Ślesak, and Agnieszka Szopa, "Significance of *Artemisia Vulgaris L.* (Common Mugwort) in the History of Medicine and Its Possible Contemporary Applications Substantiated by Phytochemical and Pharmacological Studies," *Molecules* 25, no. 19 (September 2020): 4415. *doi.org*.

44. Samuel A. Barrett and Edward W. Gifford, "Miwok Material Culture," *Bulletin of the Public Museum of the City of Milwaukee* 2, no. 4 (March 1933): 117–376. *www.yosemite.ca.us*.

45. Graeme Tobyn, Alison Denham, and Margaret Whitelegg, *The Western Herbal Tradition: 2000 Years of Medicinal Plant Knowledge* (London: Churchill Livingstone, 2010), 131.

46. Maude Grieve, *A Modern Herbal: The Medicinal, Culinary, Cosmetic and Economic Properties, Cultivation and Folklore of Herbs, Grasses, Fungi, Shrubs and Trees with All Their Modern Scientific Uses* (Paramus, NJ: Savvas Publishing, 1984, 1985).

47. Scott Camazine and Robert A. Bye, "A Study of the Medical Ethnobotany of the Zuni Indians of New Mexico," *Journal of Ethnopharmacology* 2, no. 4 (1980): 365–88.

48. James Michael Mahar, "Ethnobotany of the Oregon Paiutes of the Warm Springs Indian Reservation" (B.A. thesis, Reed College, 1953).

49. Ralph Chamberlin, *Memoirs of the American Anthropological Association, Vol. II, Part 5. The Ethno-Botany of the Gosiute Indians of Utah, pp. 331-405* (South Yarra, Victoria, Australia: Leopold Classic Library, 2016), 351.

50. Gilmore, *Some Chippewa Uses of Plants.*

51. James William Herrick, "Iroquois Medical Botany" (PhD diss., State University of New York, Albany, 1977), 498.

52. Jeffrey A. Hart, "The Ethnobotany of the Northern Cheyenne Indians of Montana," *Journal of Ethnopharmacology* 4, no. 1 (July 1981): 1–55. Here p. 27. *doi.org.*

53. John Gerard, *The Herball or Generall Historie of Plantes* (London: John Norton, 1597).

54. Isaac Jack Lévy and Rosemary Lévy Zumwalt, *Ritual Medical Lore of Sephardic Women: Sweetening the Spirits, Healing the Sick* (Champaign, IL: University of Illinois Press, 2002), 137.

55. Virgil, *The "Aeneid" of Virgil*, translated by Theodore C. Williams (Boston: Houghton Mifflin Co, 1910), Book XII.411–15. *data.perseus.org.*

56. John Brand, William Carew Hazlitt, and Henry Ellis, *Brand's Popular Antiquities of Great Britain: Faiths and Folklore; a Dictionary of National Beliefs, Superstitions, and Popular Customs, Past and Current, with Their Classical and Foreign Analogues, Described and Illustrated* (London: Reeves and Turner, 1905), 240. *catalog.hathitrust.org.*

57. Robert Tyas, *Speaking Flowers: Or Flowers to Which a Sentiment Has Been Assigned* (London: Bemrose & Sons, 1875), 91.

58. William Shakespeare, *A Midsummer Night's Dream*, Act 2, scene 1.

59. Gerard, *The Herball or Generall Historie of Plantes.*

60. Maryam Eidi, Akram Eidi, and Massih Bahar, "Effects of *Salvia officinalis L.* (Sage) Leaves on Memory Retention and Its Interaction with the Cholinergic System in Rats," *Nutrition* 22, no. 3 (March 2006): 321–26. *doi.org.*

61. Lowell John Bean and Katherine Siva Saubel, *Temalpakh (From the Earth): Cahuilla Indian Knowledge and Usage of Plants* (Banning, CA: Malki Museum Press, 1972).

62. Ken Hedges and Christina Beresford, *Santa Ysabel Ethnobotany* (San Diego: San Diego Museum of Man, 1986).

63. Richard Folkard, *Plant Lore, Legends, and Lyrics: Embracing the Myths, Traditions, Superstitions, and Folk-Lore of the Plant Kingdom* (London: Folkard & Son, 1884). *www.gutenberg.org.*

64. Shakespeare, *Hamlet*, Act 4, scene 5.

65. Grieve, *A Modern Herbal*, 682.

66. Parker L. Mott, *A Literature Review on the Status and Effects of Salvia Divinorum on Cognitive, Affective, and Behavioral Functioning* (Irvine, CA: Universal Publishers, 2011), 64.

67. Ovid, *Metamorphoses*, translated by Anthony S. Kline (2000), Bk I:525-552. *ovid.lib.virginia.edu.*

68. C. Scott Littleton, "The Pneuma Enthusiastikon: On the Possibility of Hallucinogenic 'Vapors' at Delphi and Dodona," *Ethos* 14, no. 1 (Spring 1986): 76–91. *www.jstor.org.*

69. H. H. Battles, "The Story of the Rose," *Ladies' Home Journal*, January, 1893.

70. Marie Trevelyan, *Folk-Lore and Folk-Stories of Wales* (London: Elliot Stock, 1909), 75.

71. Patricia Rain, *Vanilla: Cultural History of the World's Favorite Flavor and Fragrance* (New York: Jeremy P. Tarcher/Penguin, 2004), 124.

72. As quoted in Tim Ecott's *Vanilla: Travels in Search of the Ice Cream Orchid* (New York: Grove Press, 2005), 32.

73. John King, *King's American Dispensatory* (Cincinnati: Ohio Valley Company, 1898), 375.

74. Herodotus, *The History of Herodotus*, Book III.

75. Antony Kropff, "New English Translation of the Price Edict of Diocletianus." *www.academia.edu*, accessed February 18, 2021.

76. Hamel and Chiltoskey, *Cherokee Plants and Their Uses*, 56. Frank Speck, Royal B. Hassrick, and Edmund S. Carpenter, "Rappahannock Herbals, Folk-Lore and Science of Cures," *Proceedings of the Delaware County Institute of Science* 10 (1942): 7–55. Here p. 33.

77. Herrick, "Iroquois Medical Botany," 334.

78. Albert B. Reagan, "Plants Used by the White Mountain Apache Indians of Arizona," *The Wisconsin Archeologist*, n.s. 8 (1929): 143–61. Here p. 158. *ehrafworldcultures.yale.edu.*

79. J. Walter Fewkes, "A Contribution to Ethnobotany," *American Anthropologist* 9, no. 1 (January 1896): 14–21. Here p. 19. *doi.org.*

80. Elmore, *Ethnobotany of the Navajo.*

81. Wilfred William Robbins, John Peabody Harrington, and Barbara Freire-Marreco, "Ethnobotany of the Tewa Indians," *Bureau of American Ethnology Bulletin* 55 (1916): 1–124. Here p. 103. *repository.si.edu.*

82. Lucille J. Watahomigie and Elnora Mapatis, *Ethnobotany of the Hualapai (Hualapai Ethnobotany)* (Peach Springs, AZ: Hualapai Bilingual Program, Peach Springs School District No. 8, 1982).

83. Bean and Saubel, *Temalpakh (From the Earth).*

84. World Health Organization, "The History of Tobacco," *www.who.int,* accessed February 18, 2021.

85. Ibid.

86. Bean and Saubel, *Temalpakh (From the Earth),* 136.

87. Maurice L. Zigmond, *Kawaiisu Ethnobotany* (Salt Lake City: University of Utah Press, 1981), 43.

88. P. Leal-Galicia, D. Betancourt, A. Gonzalez-Gonzalez, and H. Romo-Parra, "A Brief History of Marijuana in the Western World," *Revista de Neurologia* 67, no. 4 (August 2018): 133–40. *pubmed.ncbi.nlm.nih.gov.*

89. Ibid.

90. Mahmoud A. ElSohly, Zlatko Mehmedic, Susan Foster, Chandrani Gon, Suman Chandra, and James C. Church, "Changes in Cannabis Potency over the Last 2 Decades (1995–2014): Analysis of Current Data in the United States," *Biological Psychiatry* 79, no. 7 (April 2016): 613–19. *doi.org.*

91. Leal-Galicia, Betancourt, Gonzalez-Gonzalez, and Romo-Parra, "A Brief History of Marijuana in the Western World."

92. Meng Ren, Zihua Tang, Xinhua Wu, Robert Spengler, Hongen Jiang, Yimin Yang, and Nicole Boivin, "The Origins of Cannabis Smoking: Chemical Residue Evidence from the First Millennium BCE in the Pamirs," *Science Advances* 5, no. 6 (June 2019). *doi.org.*

93. Eran Arie Baruch Rosen, and Dvory Namdar, "Cannabis and Frankincense at the Judahite Shrine of Arad," *Journal of the Institute of Archaeology of Tel Aviv University* 47, no. 1 (May 2020): 5–28. *doi.org.*

94. Herodotus, *The History of Herodotus,* Book 4.

95. J. R. R. Tolkien, *The Hobbit.* (Boston: Houghton Mifflin Harcourt, 2012), 1.

Bibliography

Ackerman, Diane. *A Natural History of the Senses*. New York: Knopf Doubleday Publishing Group, 2011.

Al-Harrasi, Ahmed, Abdul Latif Khan, Sajjad Asaf, and Ahmed Al-Rawahi. *Biology of Genus Boswellia*. Cham, Switzerland: Springer Nature Switzerland AG, 2019. *link.springer.com*.

Anderson, Robert, ed. *A Complete Edition of the Poets of Great Britain, Volume the Thirteenth: Containing Cook's Hesiod; Fawkes's Theocritus, Anacreon, Bion, Mosehus, Sappho, Musæus & Apollonius Rhodius; The Rape of Helen; Creech's Lucretius; and Grainger's Tibullus*. London: Arch, 1795. *books.google.com*.

Arie, Eran Baruch Rosen, and Dvory Namdar. "Cannabis and Frankincense at the Judahite Shrine of Arad." *Journal of the Institute of Archaeology of Tel Aviv University* 47, no. 1 (May 2020): 5–28. *doi.org*.

Atchley, Edward Godfrey Cuthbert Frederic. *A History of the Use of Incense in Divine Worship*. London and New York: Longmans, Green and Co., 1909.

Barrett, Samuel A., and Edward W. Gifford. "Miwok Material Culture." *Bulletin of the Public Museum of the City of Milwaukee* 2, no. 4 (March 1933): 117–376. *www.yosemite.ca.us*.

Battles, H. H. "The Story of the Rose." *Ladies' Home Journal* (January 1893).

Bean, Lowell John, and Katherine Siva Saubel. *Temalpakh (From the Earth): Cahuilla Indian Knowledge and Usage of Plants*. Banning, CA: Malki Museum Press, 1972.

Betz, Hans Dieter. *The Greek Magical Papyri in Translation: Including the Demotic Spells*. Chicago: University of Chicago Press, 1996.

Bond, Sarah. "Recreating the Aroma of the Ancient City: Incense in the Ancient Mediterranean." *Forbes*, June 26, 2017. *www.forbes.com*.

Bradford, Kevin. "The Use of Scents to Influence Consumers: The Sense of Using Scents to Make Cents." *Journal of Business Ethics* 90 (November 2009): 141–53.

Brand, John, William Carew Hazlitt, and Henry Ellis. *Brand's Popular Antiquities of Great Britain: Faiths and Folklore; a Dictionary of National Beliefs, Superstitions, and Popular Customs, Past and Current, with Their Classical and Foreign Analogues, Described and Illustrated*. London: Reeves and Turner, 1905. *catalog.hathitrust.org*.

Burr, Chandler. *The Emperor of Scent: A Story of Perfume, Obsession, and the Last Mystery of the Senses*. New York: Random House, 2003.

Camazine, Scott, and Robert A. Bye. "A Study of the Medical Ethnobotany of the Zuni Indians of New Mexico." *Journal of Ethnopharmacology* 2, no. 4 (1980): 365–88.

Chamberlin, Ralph V. *Memoirs of the American Anthropological Association, Vol. II, Part 5. The Ethno-Botany of the Gosiute Indians of Utah, pp. 331–405*. South Yarra, Victoria, Australia: Leopold Classic Library, 2016.

Clebsch, Betsy. *The New Book of Salvias: Sages for Every Garden*. Portland, OR: Timber Press, 2003.

Creasman, Pearce Paul, and Kei Yamamoto. "The African Incense Trade and Its Impacts in Pharaonic Egypt." *African Archeological Review* 36 (August 2019): 347–65. *doi.org*.

Dioscorides. *The Greek Herbal of Dioscorides*, edited by Robert T. Gunther. New York: Hafner Publishing, 1959.

Duke, James A. *Duke's Handbook of Medicinal Plants of the Bible*. Boca Raton, FL: CRC Press, 2007.

Duke, James A., and Christopher John Duke. *CRC Handbook of Medicinal Herbs*. Boca Raton, FL: CRC Press, 1985.

Ecott, Tim. *Vanilla: Travels in Search of the Ice Cream Orchid*. New York: Grove Press, 2005.

Edwards, I. E. S., C. J. Gadd, and N. G. L. Hammond, eds. *The Cambridge Ancient History*. Cambridge, UK: Cambridge University Press, 1969.

Eidi, Maryam, Akram Eidi, and Massih Bahar. "Effects of *Salvia officinalis L.* (Sage) Leaves on Memory Retention and Its Interaction with the Cholinergic System in Rats." *Nutrition* 22, no. 3 (March 2006): 321–26. *doi.org*.

Ekiert, Halina, Joanna Pajor, Paweł Klin, Agnieszka Rzepiela, Halina Ślesak, and Agnieszka Szopa. "Significance of *Artemisia Vulgaris L.* (Common Mugwort) in the History of Medicine and Its Possible Contemporary Applications Substantiated by Phytochemical and Pharmacological Studies." *Molecules* 25, no. 19 (September 2020): 4415. *doi.org*.

Elmore, Francis Hapgood. *Ethnobotany of the Navajo*. Santa Fe, NM: School of American Research, 1944. *babel.hathitrust.org*.

ElSohly, Mahmoud A., Zlatko Mehmedic, Susan Foster, Chandrani Gon, Suman Chandra, and James C. Church. "Changes in Cannabis Potency over the Last 2 Decades (1995–2014): Analysis of Current Data in the United States." *Biological Psychiatry* 79, no. 7 (April 2016): 613–19. *doi.org*.

Epstein, I., ed. *Sanhedrin Tractate*. Translated by Jacob Shachter and H. Freedman. London: Soncino Press, 1987.

Evershed, R. P., T. F. van Bergen, T. M. Peakman, E. C. Leigh-Firbank, M. C. Horton, D. Edwards, M. Biddle, B. Kjølbye-Biddle, and P. A. Rowley-Conwy. "Archaeological Frankincense." *Nature* 390 (1997): 667–68. *doi.org*.

Felter, Harvey Wickes, and John Uri Lloyd. *King's American Dispensatory*. Cincinnati: Ohio Valley Company, 1898. *www.henriettes-herb.com*.

Fewkes, J. Walter. "A Contribution to Ethnobotany." *American Anthropologist* 9, no. 1 (January 1896): 14–21. *doi.org*.

Flatt, Emma. "Spices, Smells and Spells: The Use of Olfactory Substances in the Conjuring of Spirits." *South Asian Studies* 32, no. 1 (April 2016): 3–21. *doi.org*.

Folkard, Richard. *Plant Lore, Legends, and Lyrics: Embracing the Myths, Traditions, Superstitions, and Folk-Lore of the Plant Kingdom*. London: Folkard & Son, 1884. *www.gutenberg.org*.

Geniusz, Wendy Makoons. *Our Knowledge Is Not Primitive: Decolonizing Botanical Anishinaabe Teachings (The Iroquois and Their Neighbors)*. Syracuse, NY: Syracuse University Press, 2009.

Gerard, John. *The Herball or Generall Historie of Plantes*. London: John Norton, 1597.

Gilmore, Melvin Randolph. *Some Chippewa Uses of Plants*. Ann Arbor: University of Michigan Press, 1933.

Grieve, Maude. *A Modern Herbal: The Medicinal, Culinary, Cosmetic and Economic Properties, Cultivation and Folklore of Herbs, Grasses, Fungi, Shrubs and Trees with All Their Modern Scientific Uses*. Paramus, NJ: Savvas Publishing 1984, 1985.

Halpern, Georges M., and Peter Weverka. *The Healing Trail: Essential Oils of Madagascar*. North Bergen, NJ: Basic Health Publications, 2003.

Hamel, Paul B., and Mary Ulmer Chiltoskey. *Cherokee Plants and Their Uses: A 400 Year History*. Sylva, NC: Herald Publishing Company, 1975.

Handwerk, Brian. "In Some Ways, Your Sense of Smell Is Actually Better Than a Dog's." *Smithsonian Magazine*, May 2017. *www.smithsonianmag.com*.

Hart, Jeffrey A. "The Ethnobotany of the Northern Cheyenne Indians of Montana." *Journal of Ethnopharmacology* 4, no. 1 (July 1981): 1–55. *doi.org*.

Hedges, Ken, and Christina Beresford. *Santa Ysabel Ethnobotany*. San Diego, CA: San Diego Museum of Man, 1986.

Heger, Paul. *The Development of Incense Cult in Israel*. Berlin: Walter de Gruyter, 2011.

Herodotus. *The History of Herodotus*. Translated by George Rawlinson. London: John Murray, 1858. *mit.edu*.

Herrick, James William. "Iroquois Medical Botany." PhD diss., State University of New York, Albany, 1977.

Hostetter, Aaron K., trans. "Nine Herbs Charm." Old English Poetry Project. Camden, NJ: Rutgers University, 2016. *uw.digitalmappa.org*.

Illes, Judika. *Encyclopedia of 5,000 Spells*. San Francisco: HarperOne, 2011. Kindle.

Khan, Akhtar J. "Medicinal Properties of Frankincense." *International Journal of Nutrition, Pharmacology, Neurological Diseases* 2, no. 2 (2012): 79. *www.ijnpnd.com*.

Kinkele, Thomas. *Incense and Incense Rituals*. Uttar Pradesh: B Jain Publishers Ltd., 2005.

Kotta, Sabna, Shahid H. Ansari, and Javed Ali. "Exploring Scientifically Proven Herbal Aphrodisiacs." *Pharmacognosy Review* 7, no. 13 (Jan.-Jun. 2013): 1–10. Gale Academic OneFile.

Kraft, Shelly Katheren. "Recent Changes in the Ethnobotany of Standing Rock Indian Reservation." M.A. Thesis, University of North Dakota, Grand Forks, 1990.

Kropff, Antony. "New English Translation of the Price Edict of Diocletianus." *www.academia.edu.* Accessed February 18, 2021.

Leal-Galicia, P., D. Betancourt, A. Gonzalez-Gonzalez, and H. Romo-Parra. "A Brief History of Marijuana in the Western World." *Revista de Neurologia* 67, no. 4 (August 2018): 133–40. *pubmed.ncbi.nlm.nih.gov.*

Lemenih, Mulugeta, and Demel Teketay. "Frankincense and Myrrh Resources of Ethiopia: II. Medicinal and Industrial Uses." *SINET: Ethiopian Journal of Science* 26, no. 2 (2003): 161–72. *semanticscholar.org.*

Lévy, Isaac Jack, and Rosemary Lévy Zumwalt. *Ritual Medical Lore of Sephardic Women: Sweetening the Spirits, Healing the Sick.* Champaign, IL: University of Illinois Press, 2002.

Littleton, C. Scott. "The Pneuma Enthusiastikon: On the Possibility of Hallucinogenic 'Vapors' at Delphi and Dodona." *Ethos* 14, no. 1 (Spring 1986): 76–91. *www.jstor.org.*

Mahar, James Michael. "Ethnobotany of the Oregon Paiutes of the Warm Springs Indian Reservation." B.A. Thesis, Reed College, 1953.

Mäkinen, Martti. "Henry Daniel's Rosemary in MS X.90 of the Royal Library, Stockholm." *Neuphilologische Mitteilungen* 103, no. 3 (2002): 305–27. *www.jstor.org.*

Manniche, Lise. *Sacred Luxuries: Fragrance, Aromatherapy, and Cosmetics in Ancient Egypt.* Ithaca, NY: Cornell University Press, 1999.

McPartland, John M., William Hegman, and Tengwen Long. "*Cannabis* in Asia: Its Center of Origin and Early Cultivation, Based on a Synthesis of Subfossil Pollen and Archaeobotanical Studies." *Vegetation History and Archaeobotany* 28 (2019): 691–702. *doi.org.*

Miller, Richard Alan, and Iona Miller. *The Magical and Ritual Use of Perfumes.* Rochester, VT: Destiny Books, 1990.

Morgan, Jamie. "Womb with a View: Sensory Development in Utero." *UT Southwestern Medical Center*, August 1, 2017. *utswmed.org.*

Mott, Parker L. *A Literature Review on the Status and Effects of Salvia Divinorum on Cognitive, Affective, and Behavioral Functioning.* Irvine, CA: Universal Publishers, 2011.

Munro, John. "The Consumption of Spices and Their Costs in Late-Medieval and Early-Modern Europe: Luxuries or Necessities?" Lecture, University of Toronto, November 8, 1988. *www.economics.utoronto.ca.*

Nemu, Danny. "Getting High with the Most High: Entheogens in the Old Testament." *Journal of Psychedelic Studies* 3, no. 2 (2019). *doi.org*.

Nicholson, Paul T., and Ian Shaw, eds. *Ancient Egyptian Materials and Technology*. Cambridge, UK: Cambridge University Press, 2000.

Nielsen, Kjeld. *Incense in Ancient Israel*. Leiden, The Netherlands: Brill Academic Publishing, 2014.

Odin (human author unknown). Nine Herbs Charm. Mid-10th century. Translated by Wikisource. *en.wikisource.org*.

Ovid. *Metamorphoses*. Translated by Anthony S. Kline, 2000. *ovid.lib.virginia.edu*.

Peacock, David, and David Williams. *Food for the Gods: New Light on the Ancient Incense Trade*. Oxford: Oxbow Books, 2006. Kindle.

Peter, K.V., ed. *Handbook of Herbs and Spices: Volume 3*. Cambridge, UK: Woodhead Publishing, 2006.

Preisendanz, Karl. *Papyri Graecae Magicae, Volume 1*. Leipzig, Germany: Teubner, 1928. *doi.org*.

Rain, Patricia. *Vanilla: Cultural History of the World's Favorite Flavor and Fragrance*. New York: Jeremy P. Tarcher/Penguin, 2004.

Reagan, Albert B. "Plants Used by the White Mountain Apache Indians of Arizona." *The Wisconsin Archeologist*, n.s. 8 (1929): 143–61. *ehrafworldcultures.yale.edu*.

Ren, Meng, Zihua Tang, Xinhua Wu, Robert Spengler, Hongen Jiang, Yimin Yang, and Nicole Boivin. "The Origins of Cannabis Smoking: Chemical Residue Evidence from the First Millennium BCE in the Pamirs." *Science Advances* 5, no. 6 (June 2019). *doi.org*.

Robbins, Wilfred William, John Peabody Harrington, and Barbara Freire-Marreco. "Ethnobotany of the Tewa Indians." *Bureau of American Ethnology Bulletin* 55 (1916): 1–124. *repository.si.edu*.

Rollason, David. *Early Medieval Europe 300–1050: A Guide for Studying and Teaching*. second edition (London: Routledge, 2018).

Rousseau, Jacques, 1945. "Le Folklore Botanique De Caughnawaga." *Contributions de l'Institut botanique l'Universite de Montreal* 55 (1945): 7–72.

Sayorwan, Winai, Nijsiri Ruangrungsi, Teerut Piriyapunyporn, Tapnee Hongratanaworakit, Naiphinich Kotchabhakdi, and Vorasith Siriporn-panich. "Effects of Inhaled Rosemary Oil on Subjective Feelings and

Activities of the Nervous System." *Scientia Pharmaceutica* 81, no. 2 (April-June 2013): 531–42.

Schultz, Colin. "There's More to Frankincense and Myrrh Than Meets the Eye." *Smithsonian Magazine*, December 24, 2014. *www.smithsonianmag.com.*

Sell, C. S. *Chemistry and the Sense of Smell*. Hoboken, NJ: Wiley. 2014.

Shakespeare, William. *Hamlet*. Edited by Barbara A. Mowat and Paul Werstine. New York: Simon & Schuster, 1992.

———. *A Midsummer Night's Dream*. Boston: Ginn and Company, 1910.

Shichida, Yoshinori, Takahiro Yamashita, Hiroo Imai, and Takushi Kishida. *Evolution and Senses: Opsins, Bitter Taste, and Olfaction*. New York: Springer, 2013.

Smith, Huron H. "Ethnobotany of the Forest Potawatomi Indians." *Bulletin of the Public Museum of the City of Milwaukee* 7 (1933): 1–230.

Smith-Williams, Henry. *The Historians' History of the World: A Comprehensive Narrative of the Rise and Development of Nations from the Earliest Times*, Volumes 1–2. Encyclopaedia Britannica, 1907.

Sowndhararajan, Kandhasamy, and Songmun Kim. "Influence of Fragrances on Human Psychophysiological Activity: With Special Reference to Human Electroencephalographic Response." *Scientia Pharmaceutica* 84, no. 4 (November 2016): 724–51. *doi.org.*

Speck, Frank F., Royal B. Hassrick, and Edmund S. Carpenter. "Rappahannock Herbals, Folk-Lore and Science of Cures." *Proceedings of the Delaware County Institute of Science* 10 (1942): 7–55.

Stoddart, David Michael. *The Scented Ape: The Biology and Culture of Human Odour*. Cambridge, UK: Cambridge University Press, 1990.

Strebel, Danielle M., Andrew J. Fangel, Tony M. Wolfe, and Emily J. Mason. "Anxiolytic and Anti-Depressant Effects of *Boswellia* Extract on CD1 *Mus musculus*." *BIOS* 85, no. 2 (May 2014): 79–85. *doi.org.*

Tobyn, Graeme, Alison Denham, and Margaret Whitelegg. *The Western Herbal Tradition: 2000 Years of Medicinal Plant Knowledge*. London: Churchill Livingstone, 2010.

Trevelyan, Marie. *Folk-Lore and Folk-Stories of Wales*. London: Elliot Stock, 1909.

Turin, Luca. *The Secret of Scent: Adventures in Perfume and the Science of Smell*. New York: Harper Perennial, 2007.

Tyas, Robert. *Speaking Flowers: Or Flowers to Which a Sentiment Has Been Assigned*. London: Bemrose & Sons, 1875.

Tyson, Peter. "Dogs' Dazzling Sense of Smell." *Nova*, October 4, 2012. *www.pbs.org.*

Van Beek, Gus W. "Frankincense and Myrrh in Ancient South Arabia." *Journal of the American Oriental Society* 78, no. 3 (July-September 1958): 141–52. *www.jstor.org.*

Vestal, Paul A., and Richard Evans Schultes. *The Economic Botany of the Kiowa Indians: As It Relates to the History of the Tribe*. Cambridge, MA: Botanical Museum, 1939. *hdl.handle.net.*

Virgil. *The "Aeneid" of Virgil*. Translated by Theodore C. Williams. Boston: Houghton Mifflin Co, 1910. *data.perseus.org.*

Watahomigie, Lucille J., and Elnora Mapatis. *Ethnobotany of the Hualapai (Hualapai Ethnobotany)*. Peach Springs, AZ: Hualapai Bilingual Program, Peach Springs School District No. 8, 1982.

Watt, Martin, and Wanda Sellar. *Frankincense and Myrrh: Through the Ages and a Complete Guide to Their Use in Herbalism and Aromatherapy Today*. London: Ebury Publishing, 2012.

Watts, D. C. *Dictionary of Plant Lore*. Cambridge, MA: Academic Press, 2007.

Wildwood, Chrissie. *Mood Enhancing Plants*. London: Ebury Publishing, 2011.

Williams, Henry Smith. *The Historians' History of the World: A Comprehensive Narrative of the Rise and Development of Nations from the Earliest Times, Volumes 1-2*. London: Encyclopaedia Britannica Co. Ltd., 1926.

World Health Organization. "The History of Tobacco." *www.who.int.* Accessed February 18, 2021.

Zigmond, Maurice L. *Kawaiisu Ethnobotany*. Salt Lake City: University of Utah Press, 1981

Index

ABOUT THE AUTHOR

SARA L. MASTROS holds a master's degree in theoretical mathematics and was a high school and college teacher for nearly a decade before quitting to practice witchcraft full time. She is co-owner of Mastros and Zealot, where she offers custom sorcery, courses on practical magic, and has for many years made and sold magical incense online and at Pagan and occult festivals all over the East Coast. Mastros has been a contributor to *Witches & Pagans*, *Cartomancer*, and other magazines. The second edition of her first book, *Orphic Hymns Grimoire*, is forthcoming from Hadean Press. She is also the co-owner and chief content officer of Quicksilver Cards and Games, who produce (among other apps), the bestselling line of Fool's Dog tarot apps.

To Our Readers